Jazz Classics

Amsco Publications
New York • London • Sydney

This book Copyright © 1996 by Amsco Publications,
A Division of Music Sales Corporation, New York

All Rights Reserved. No part of this publication may be reproduced
by in any form or by any electronic or mechanical means, including
information storage and retrieval systems, without permission in
writing from the publisher.

Order No. AM 934373
US International Standard Book Number: 0.8256.1529.1
UK International Standard Book Number: 0.7119.5406.2

Exclusive Distributors:
Music Sales Corporation
257 Park Avenue South, New York, NY 10010 USA
Music Sales Limited
8/9 Frith Street, London W1V 5TZ England
Music Sales Pty. Limited
120 Rothschild Avenue, Rosebery, NSW 2018, Australia

Printed in the United States of America by
Vicks Lithograph and Printing Corporation

Allen's Alley *26*

Anthropology *4*

Blood Count *58*

Bouncin' With Bud *28*

Epistrophy *31*

52nd Street Theme *6*

In Walked Bud *10*

Jersey Bounce *62*

Ladybird *34*

Lush Life *48*

Manteca *36*

Monk's Mood *18*

Off Minor *44*

Oop Bop Sh' Bam *46*

Perdido *13*

Ruby, My Dear *16*

Shaw Nuff *52*

Soul Sauce *24*

Tempus Fugit *56*

Thelonious *39*

Two Bass Hit *21*

Wouldn't You *42*

Anthropology

by Dizzy Gillespie and Charles Parker

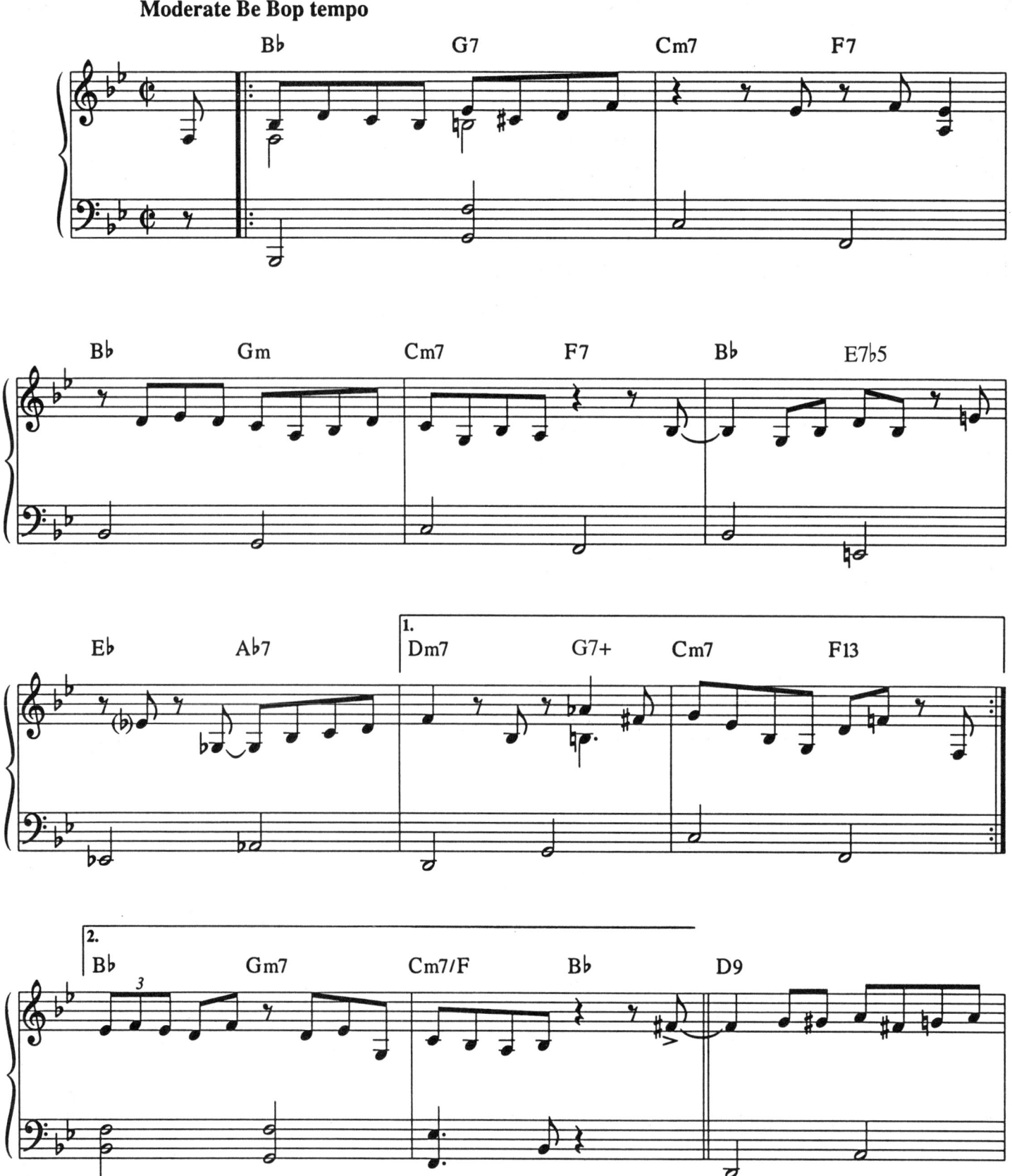

Copyright © 1948 (Renewed) by Music Sales Corporation (ASCAP) and Criterion Music Corp.
International Copyright Secured. All Rights Reserved.

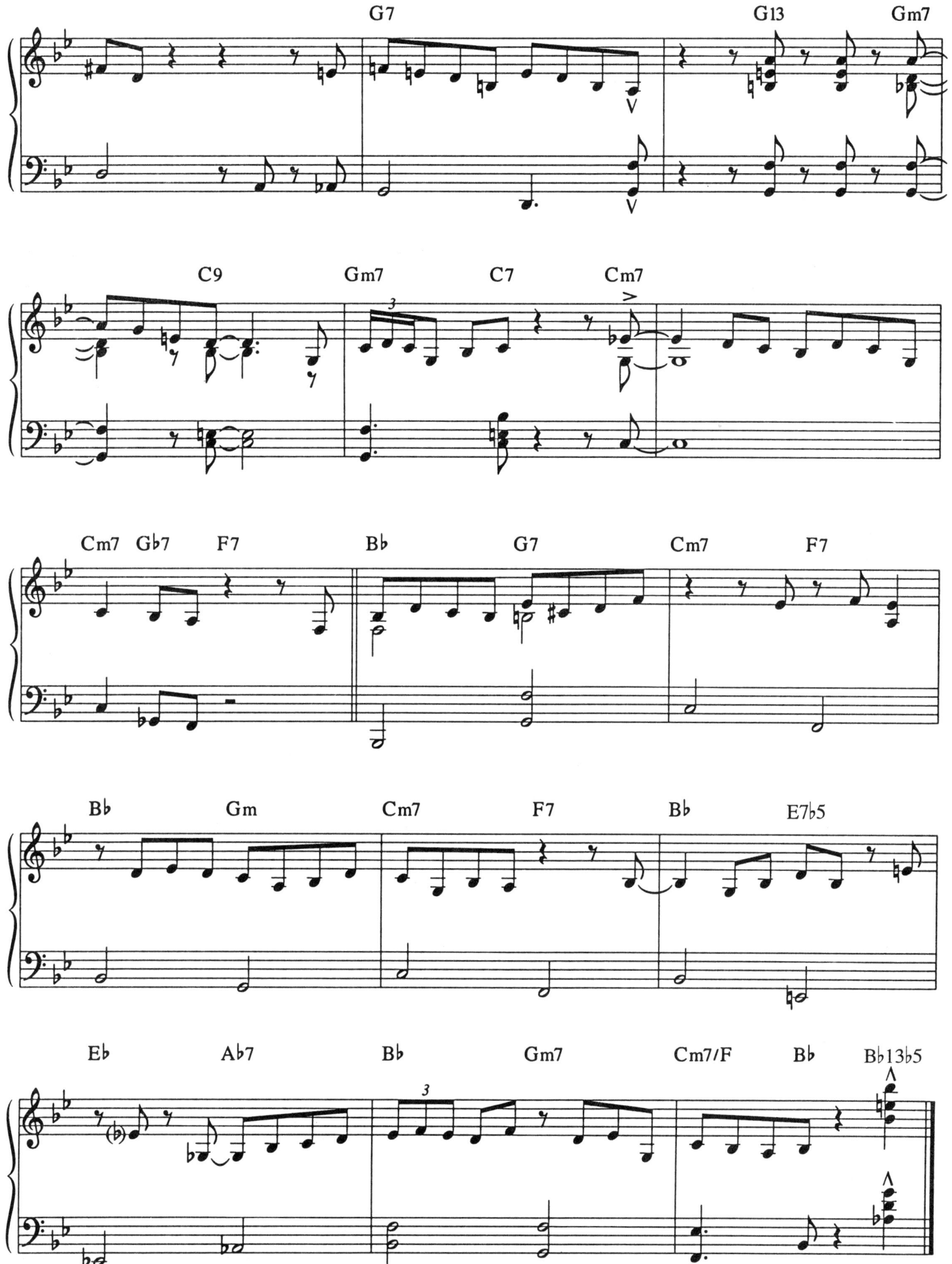

52nd Street Theme
by Thelonious Monk

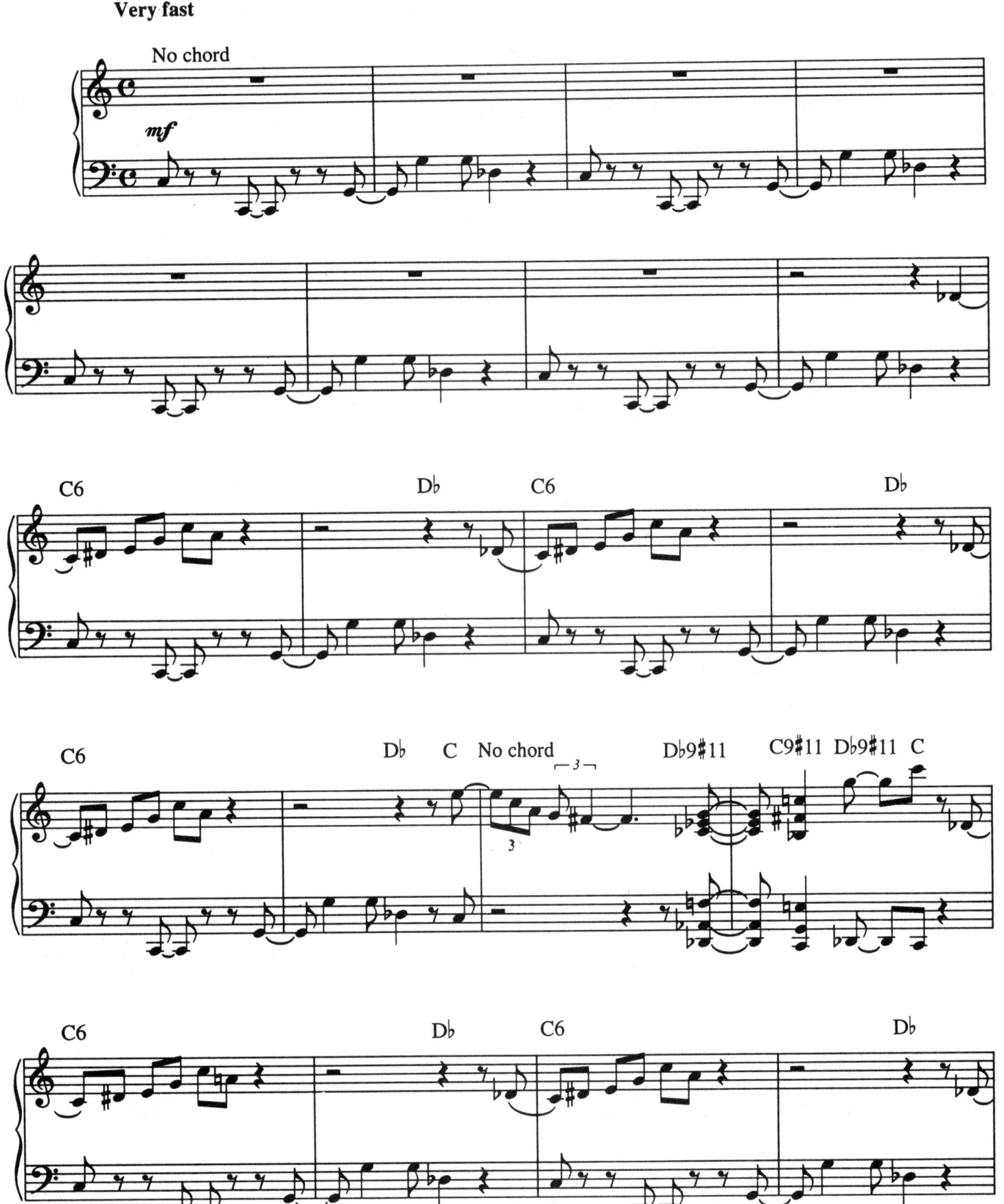

Copyright © 1944 (Renewed) by Music Sales Corporation (ASCAP) and Embassy Music Corporation (BMI)
International Copyright Secured. All Rights Reserved.

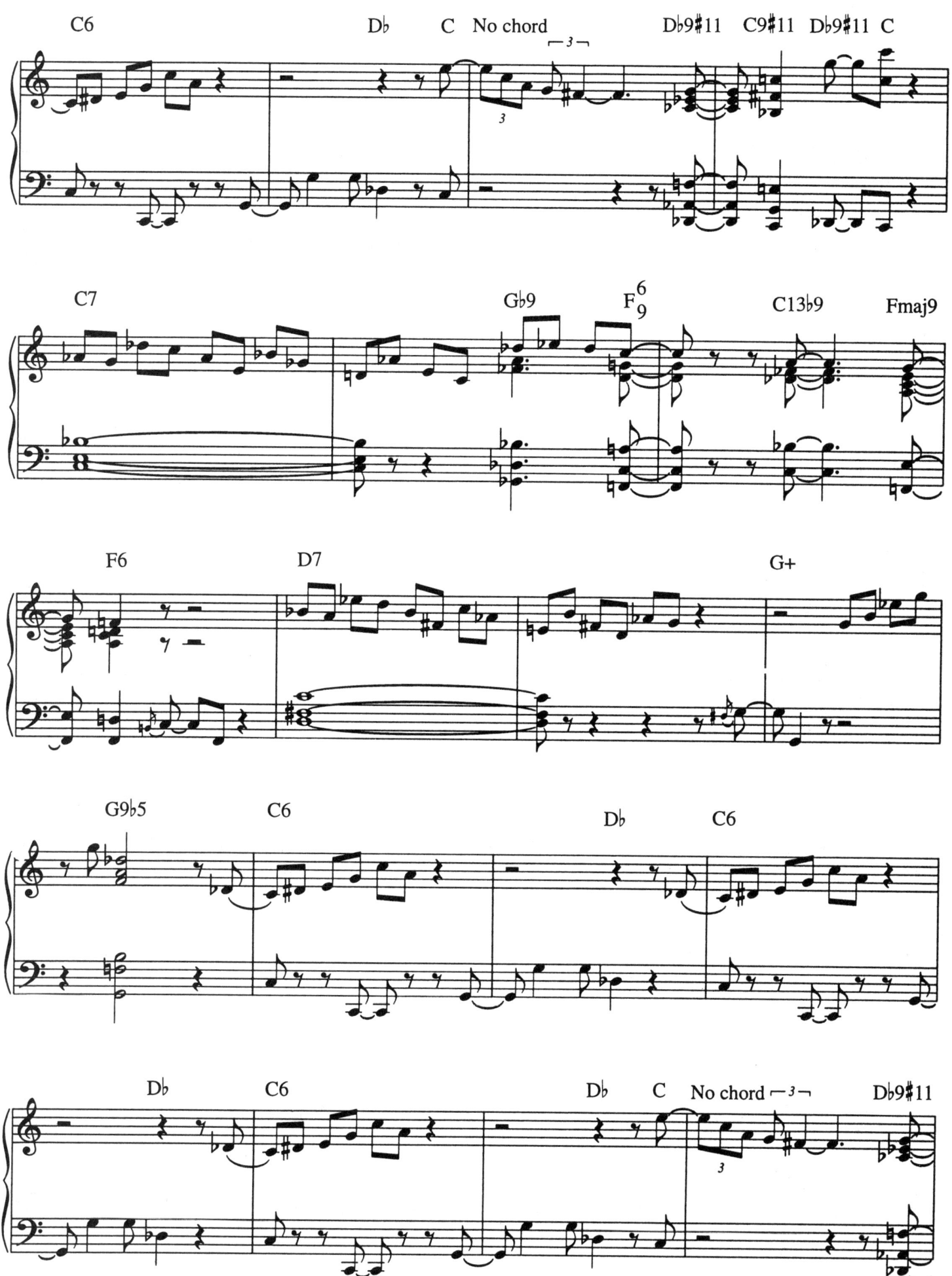

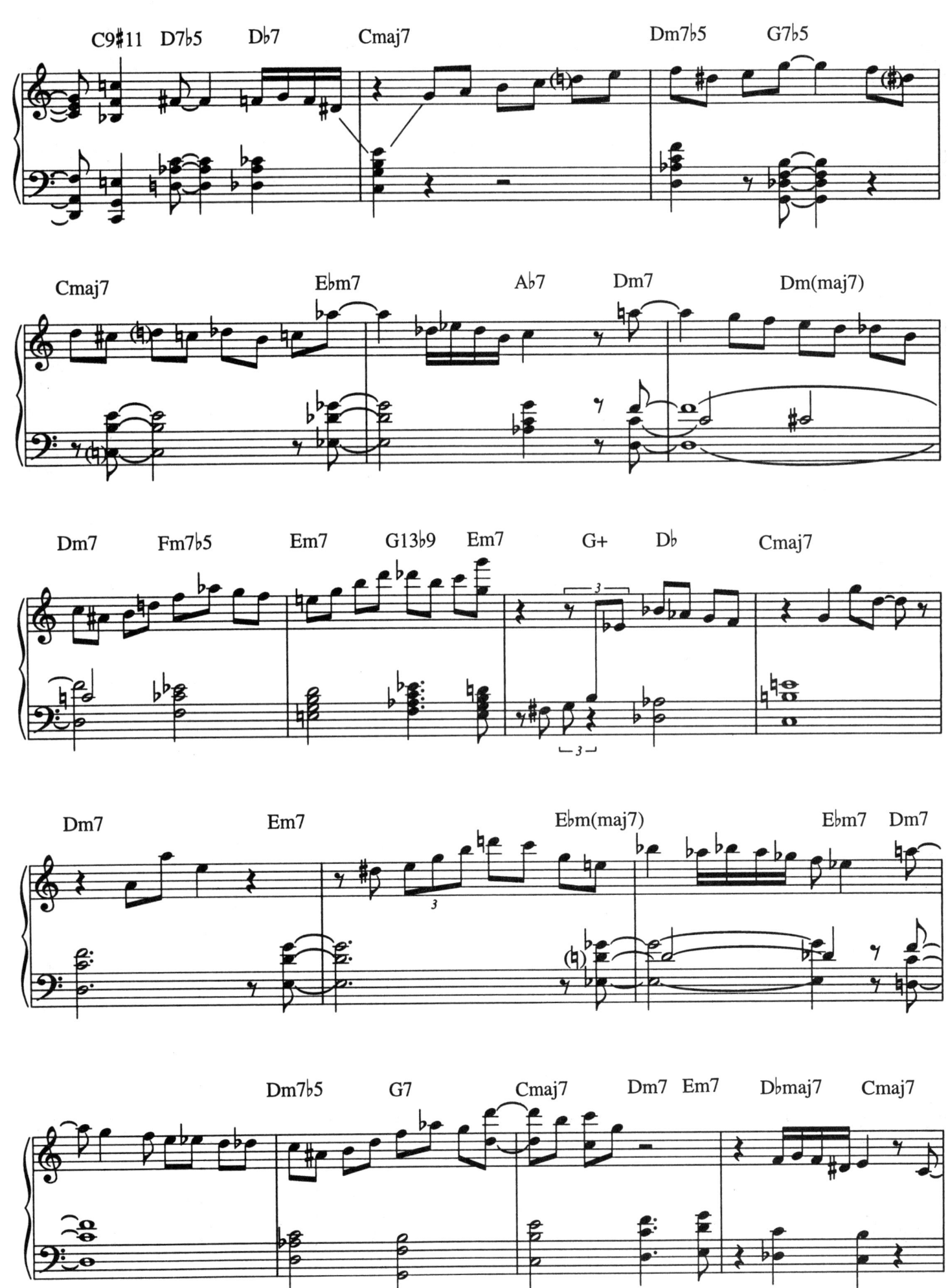

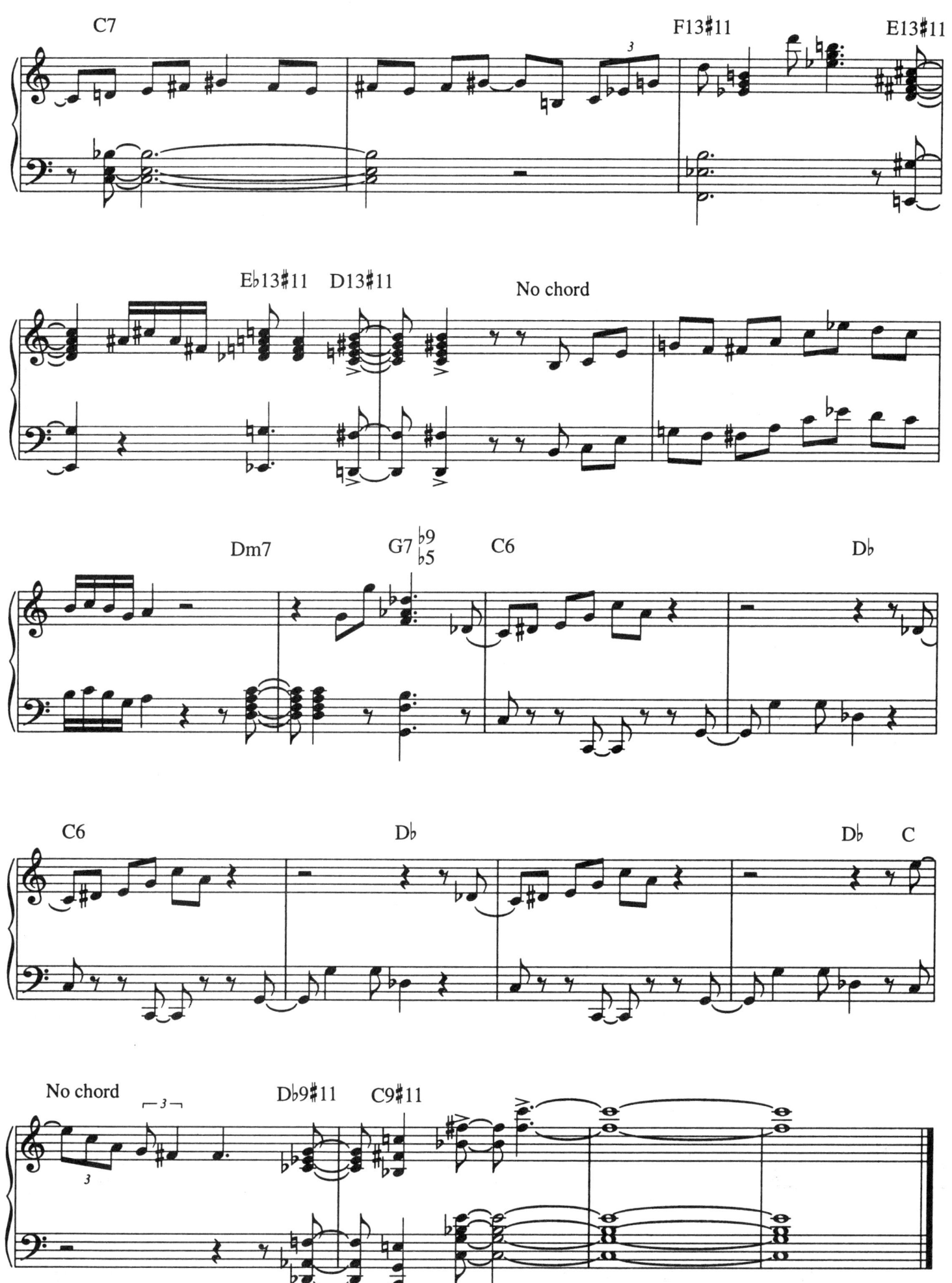

In Walked Bud

by Thelonious Monk

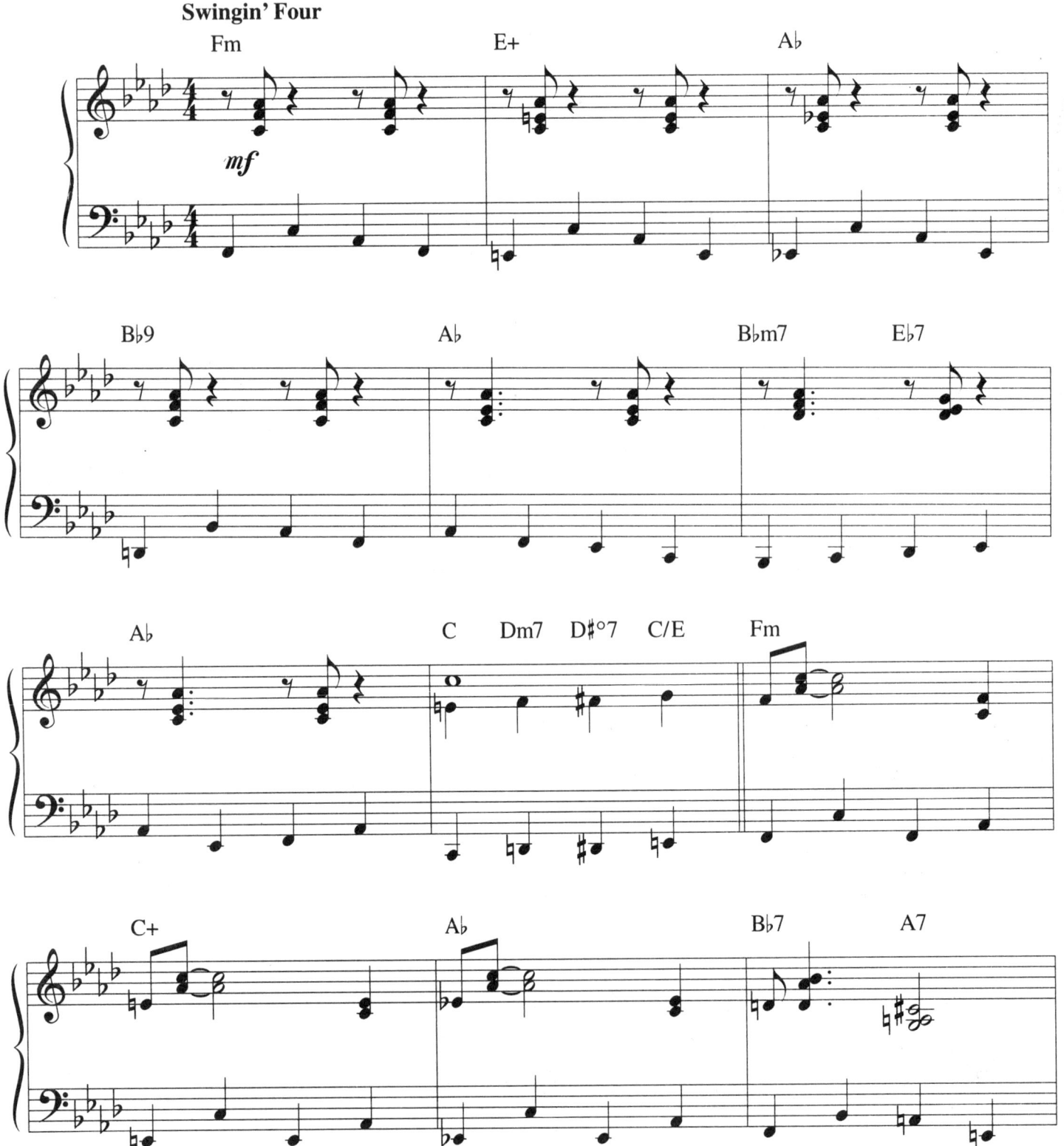

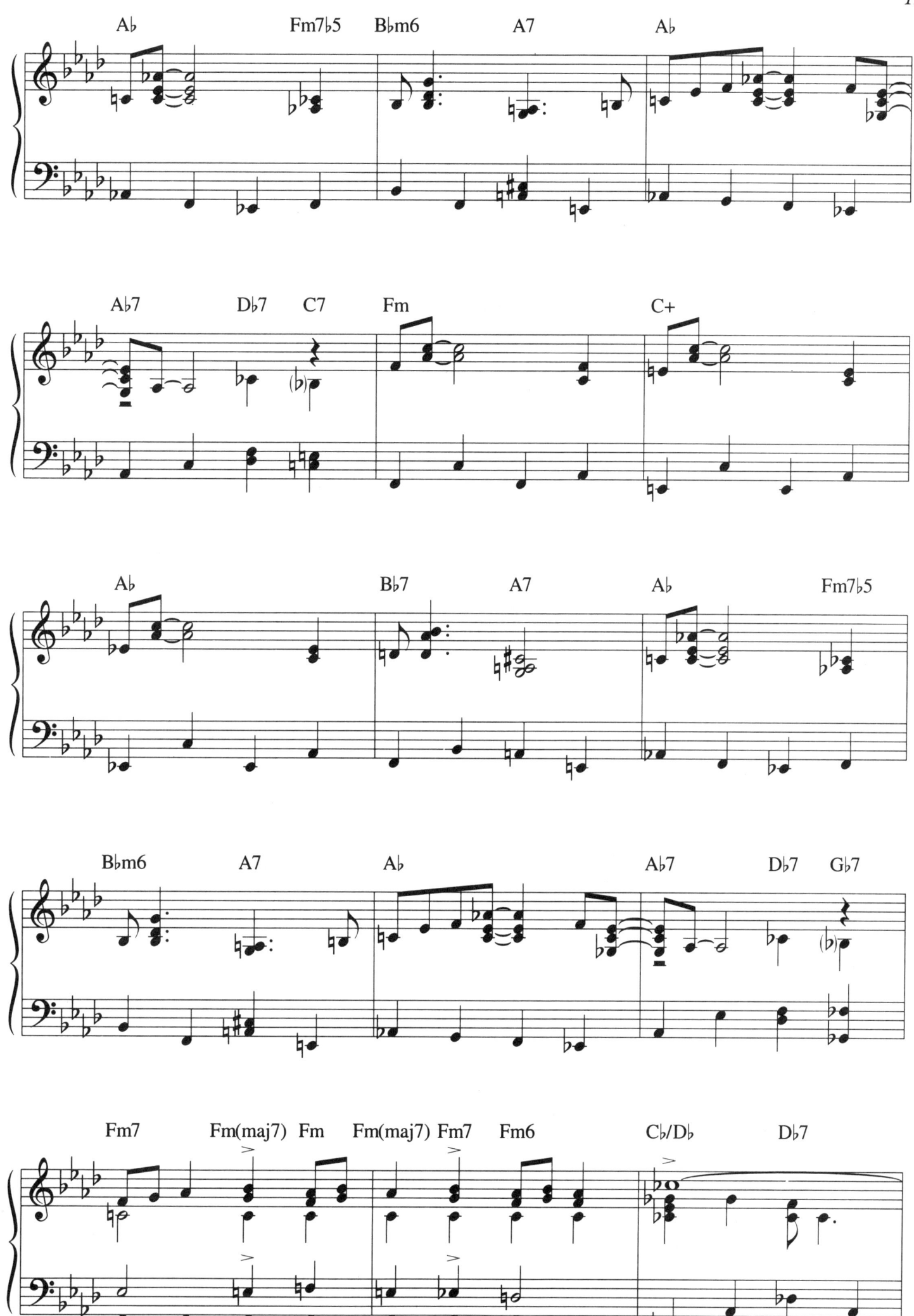

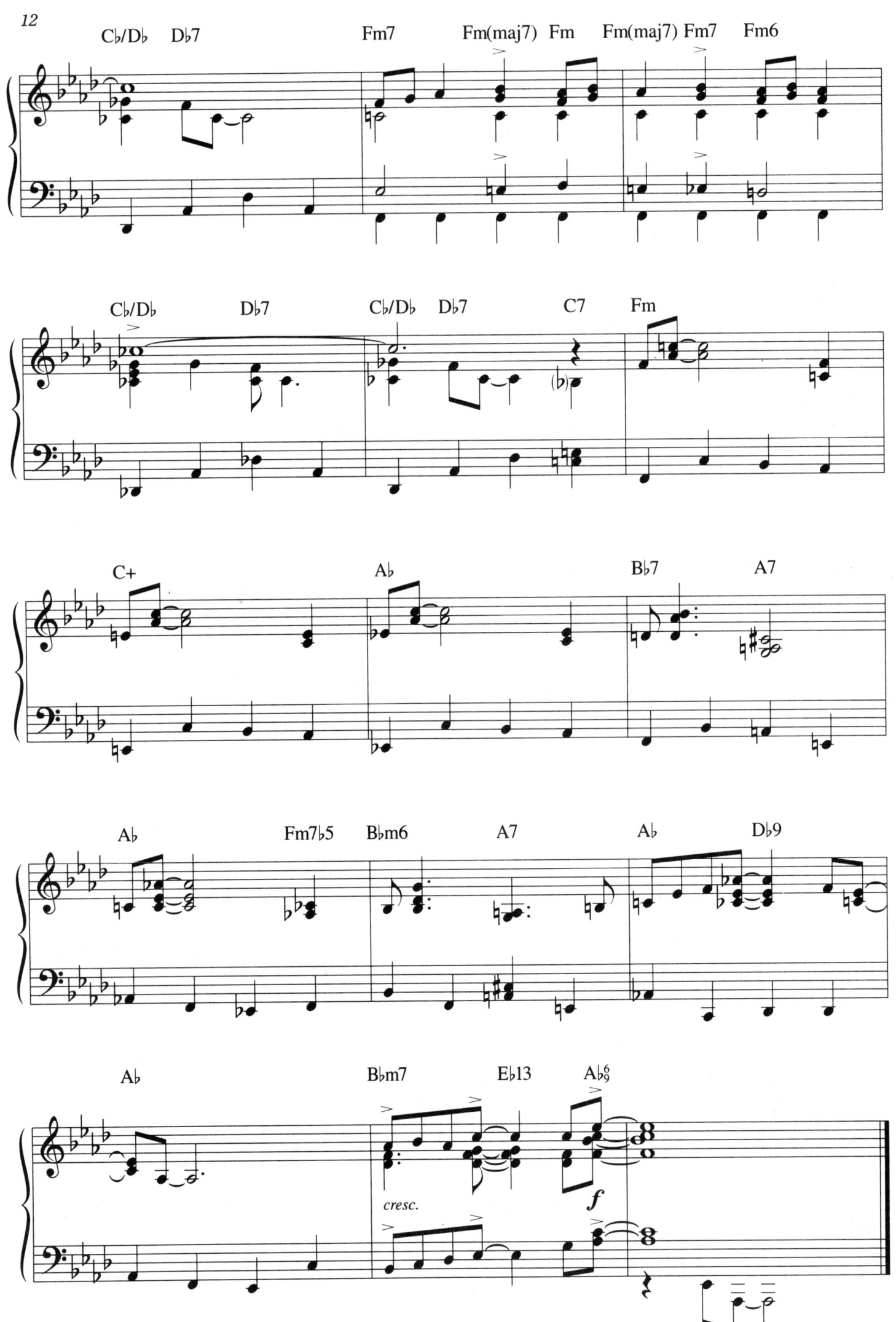

Perdido

by Juan Tizol

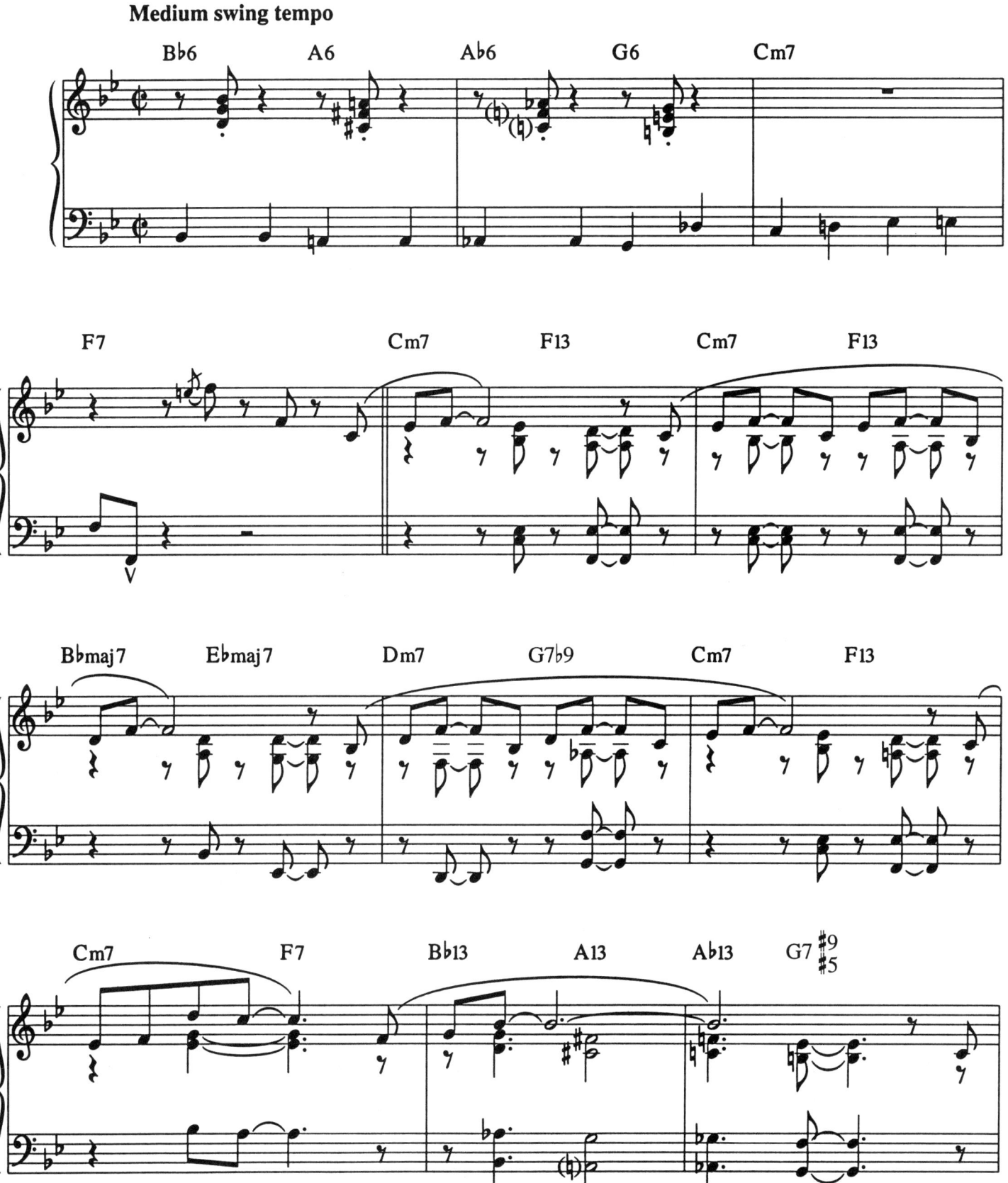

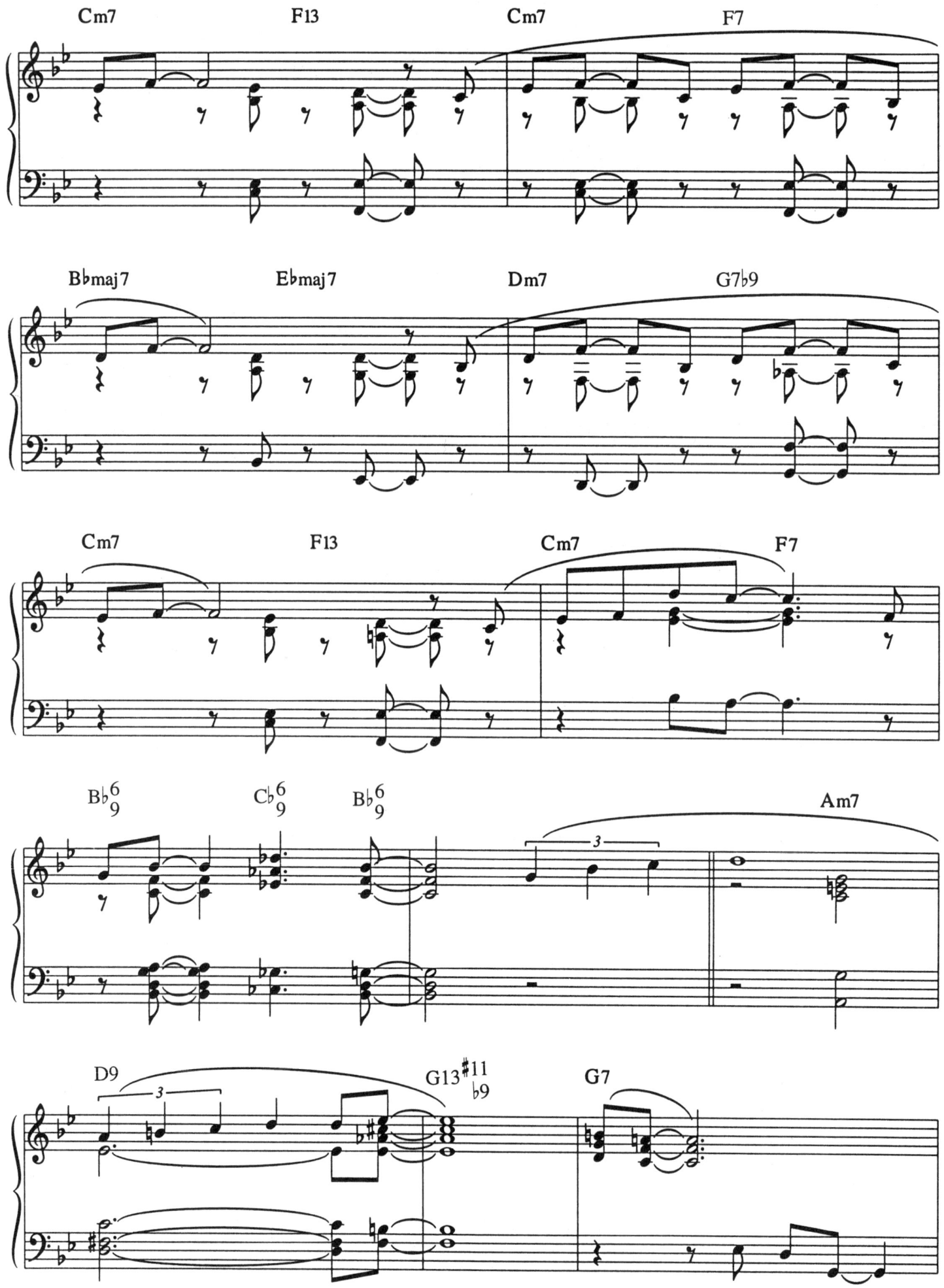

Gm7/C
C9
3
Cm9
G13
G♭13
F13
Cm7
F13
Cm7
F13
B♭maj7
E♭maj7
Dm7
G7♭9
Cm7
F13
Cm7
F13
A♭13
A13
B♭6/9
B♭13 #9 ♭5

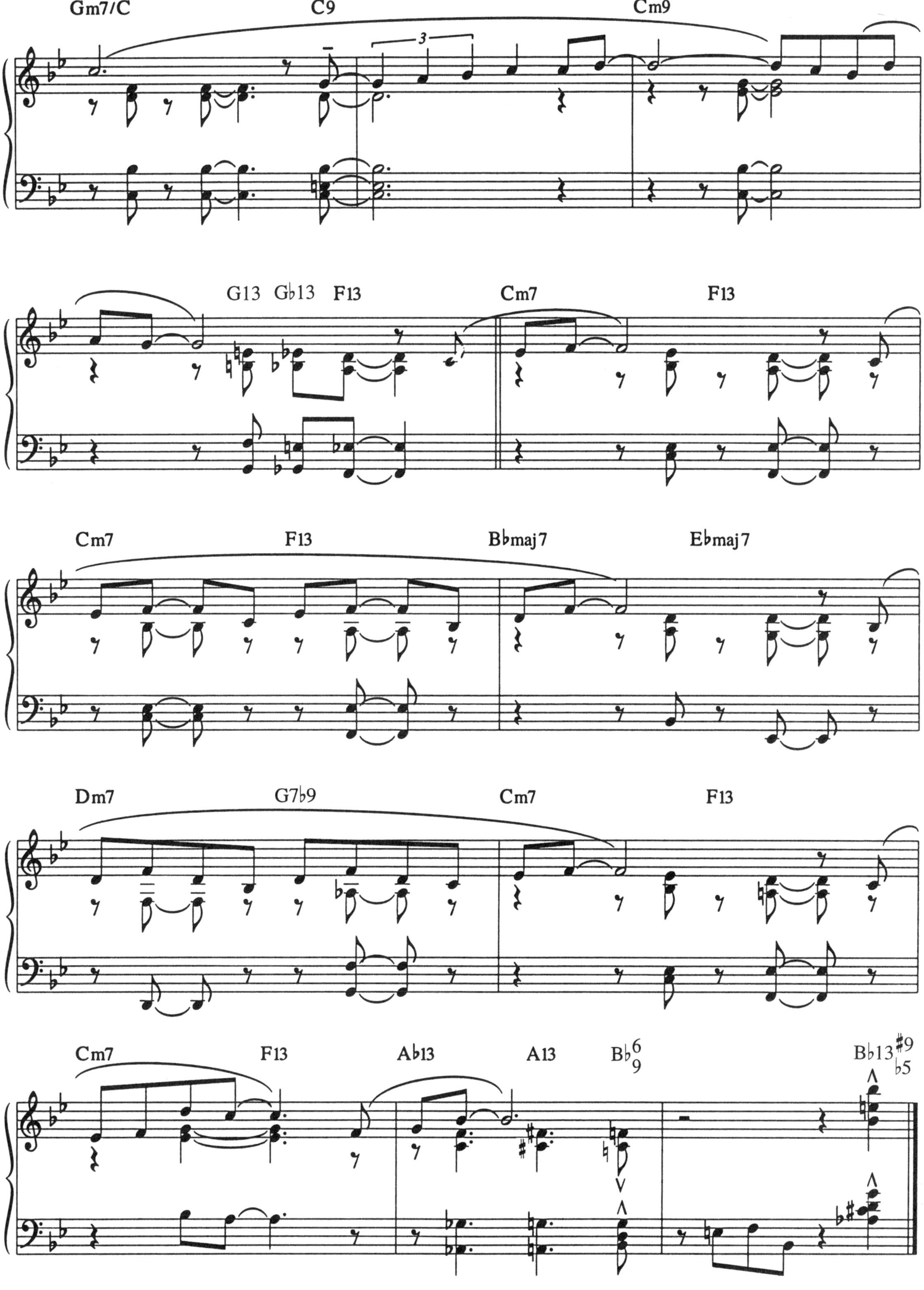

Ruby, My Dear

by Thelonious Monk

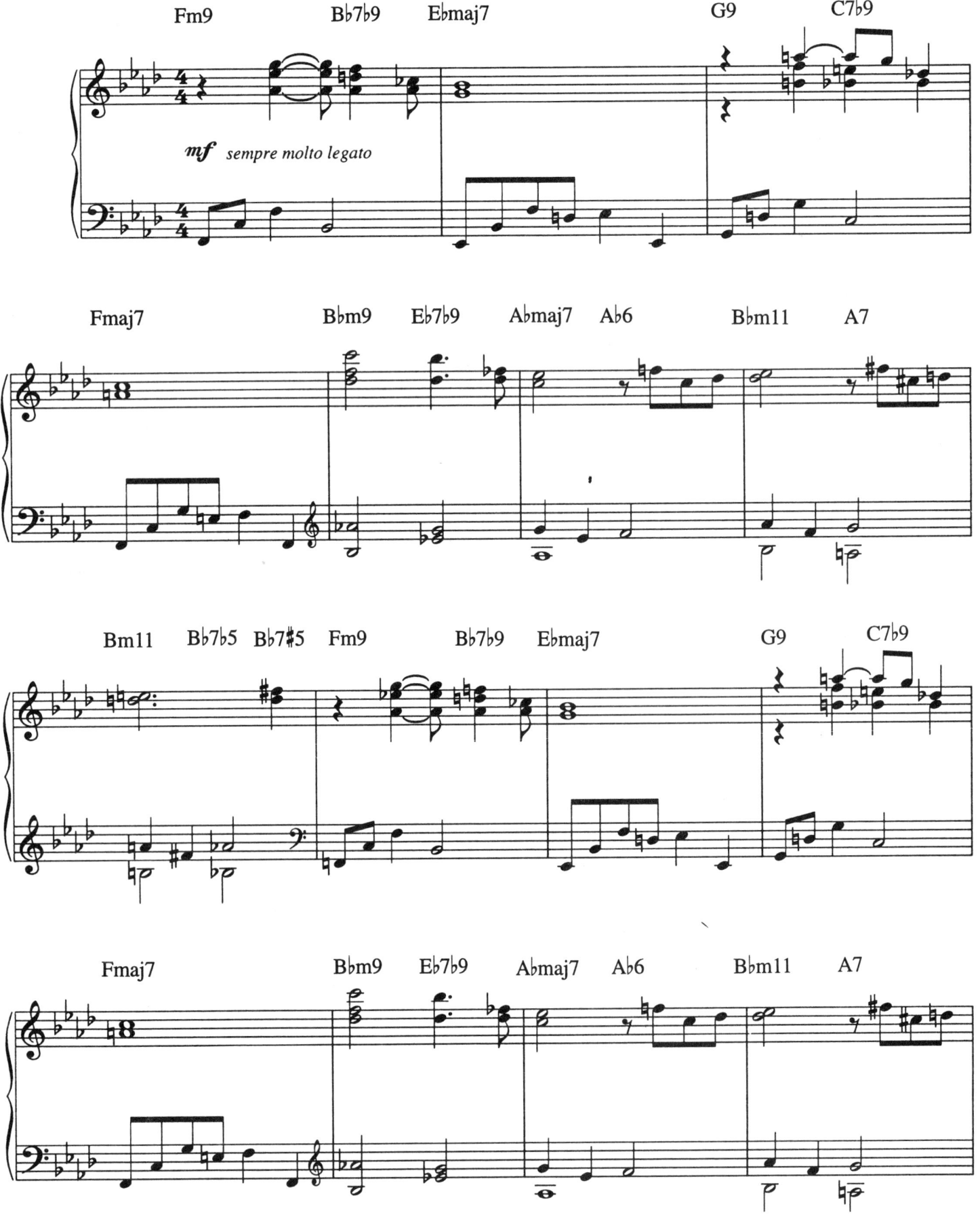

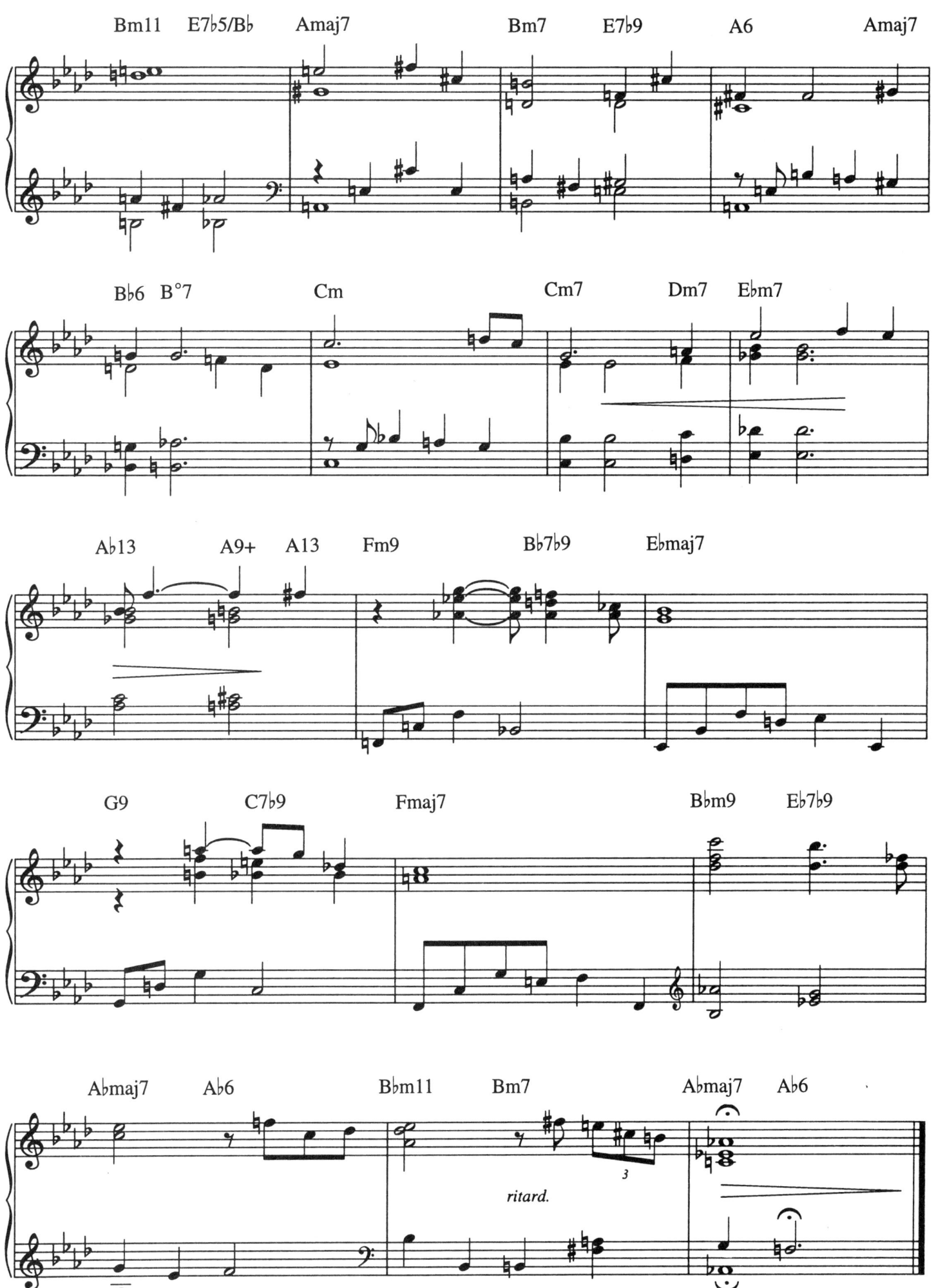

Monk's Mood
(a/k/a Feeling That Way Now)
by Thelonious Monk

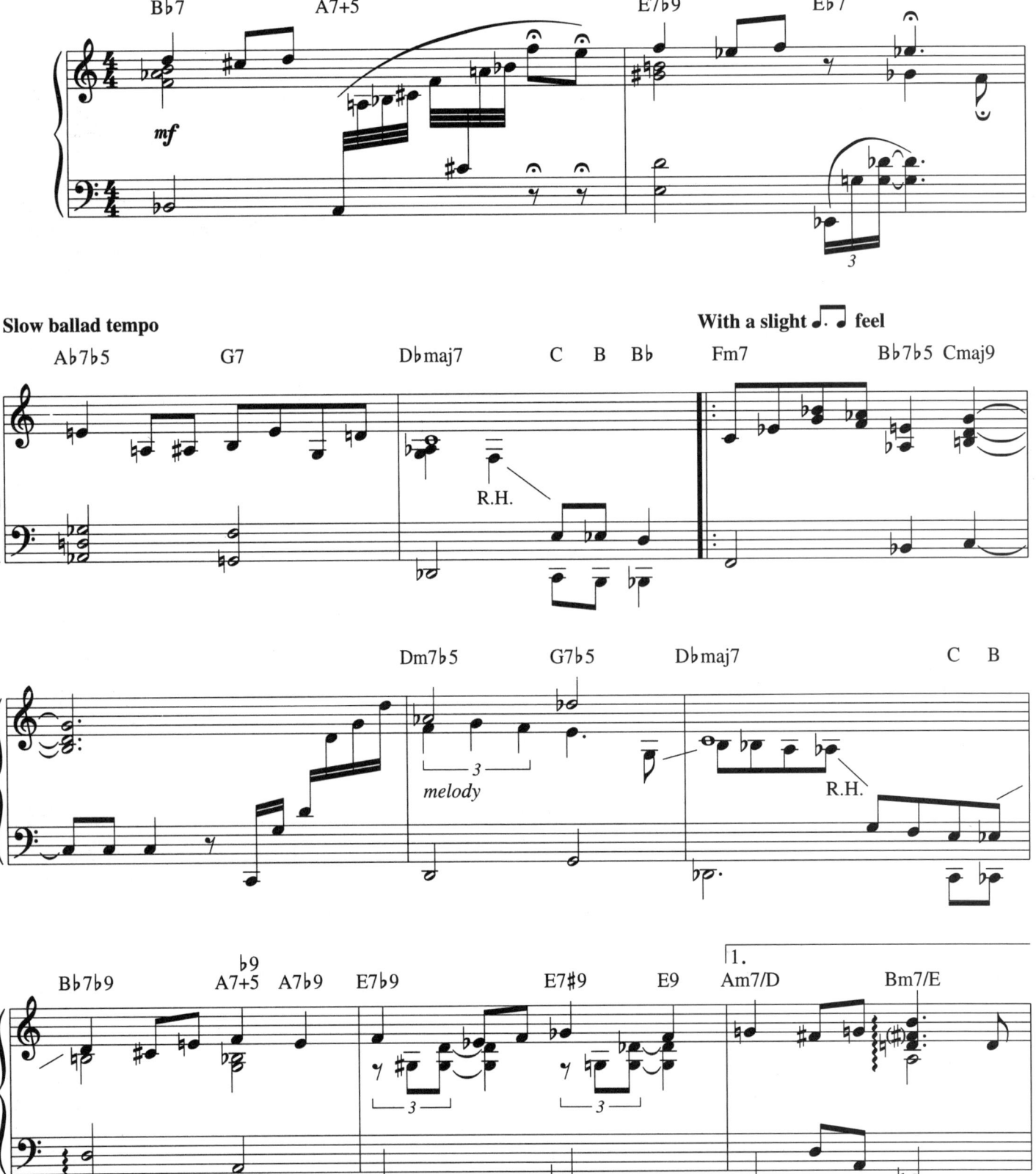

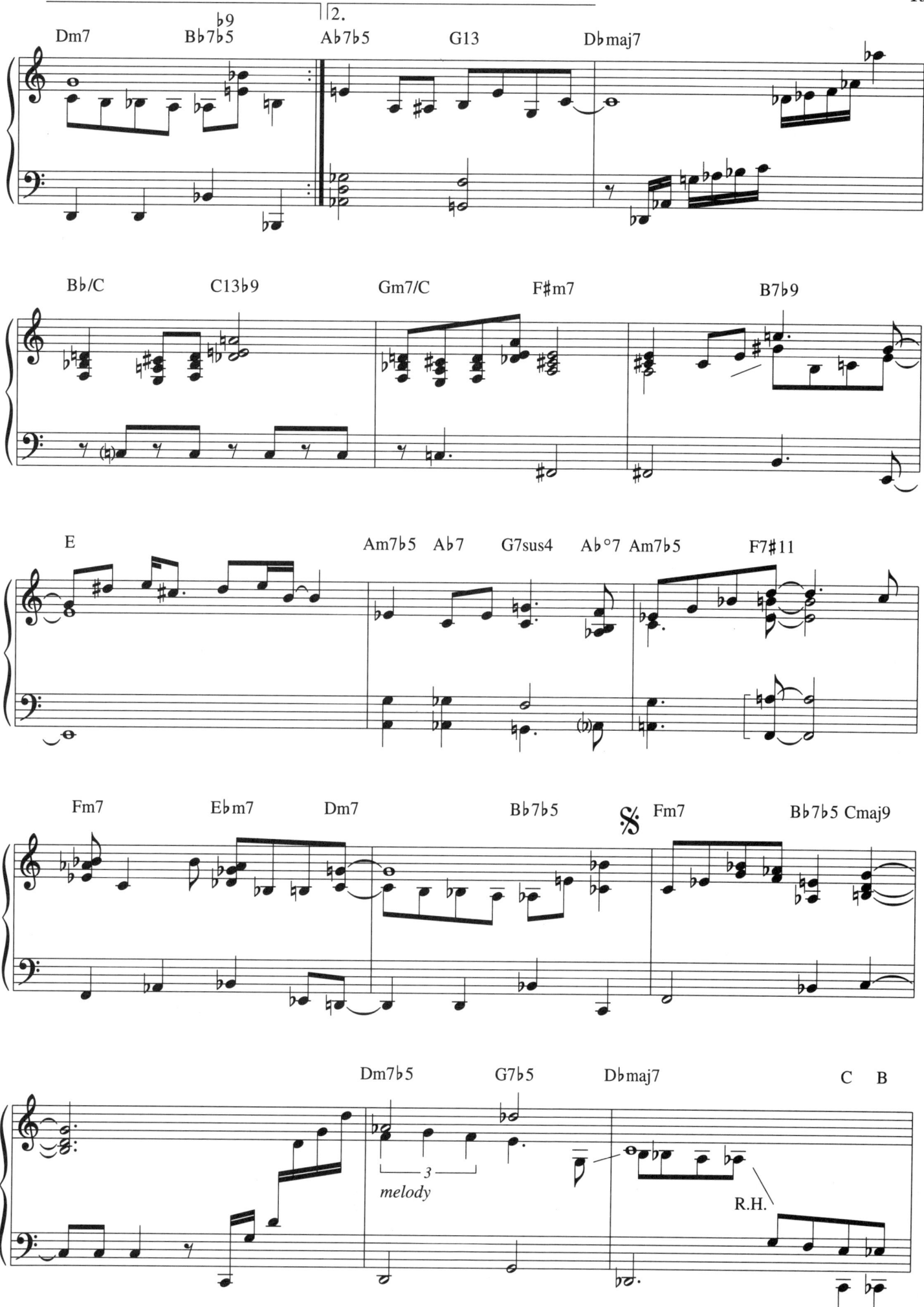

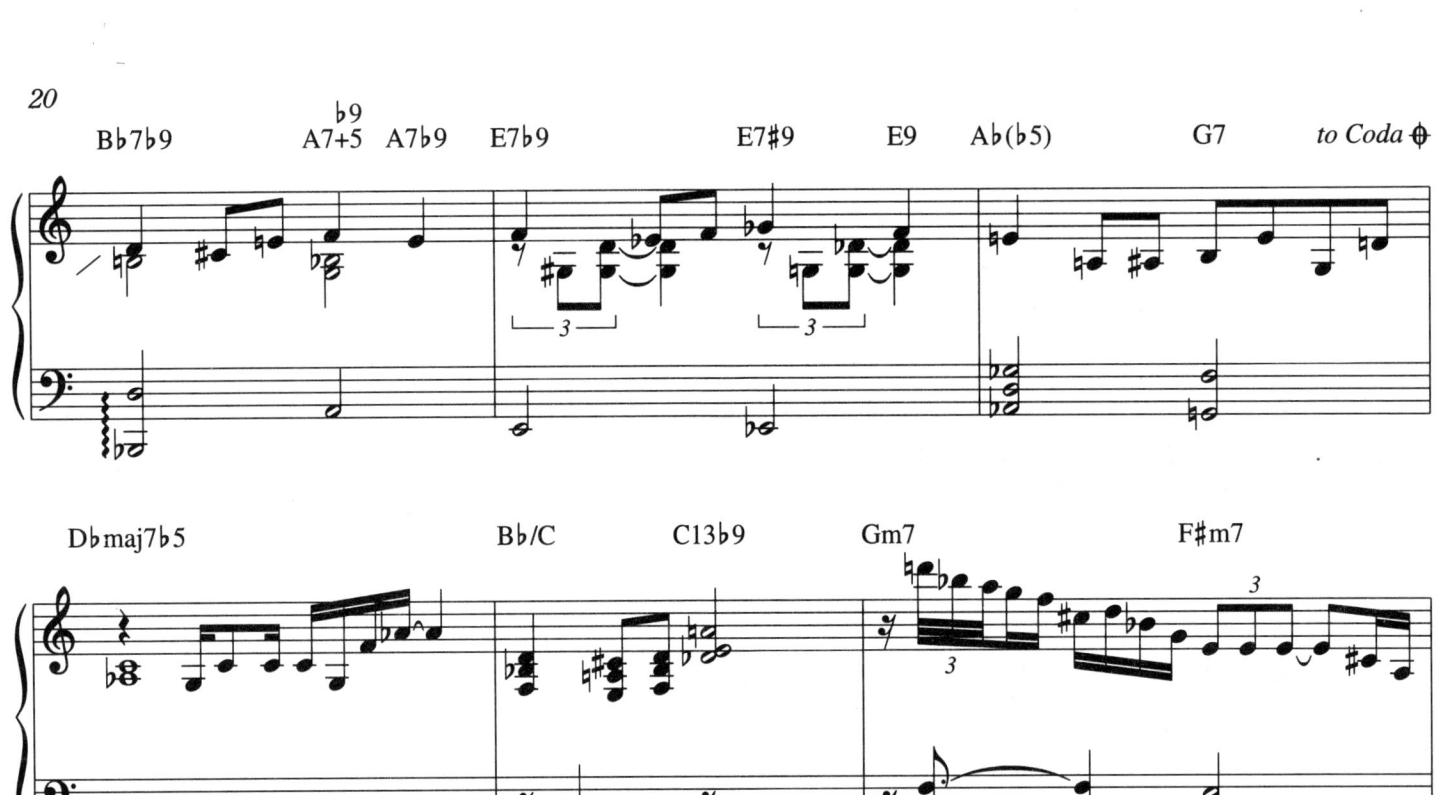
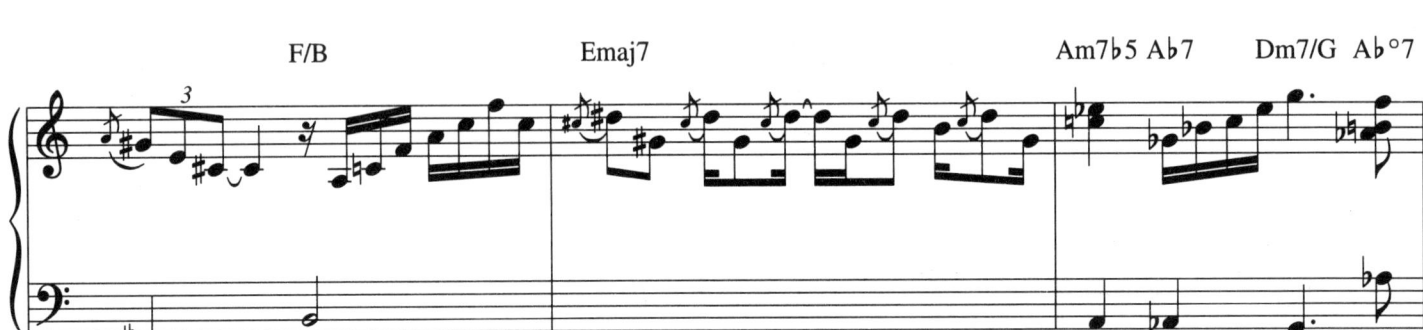
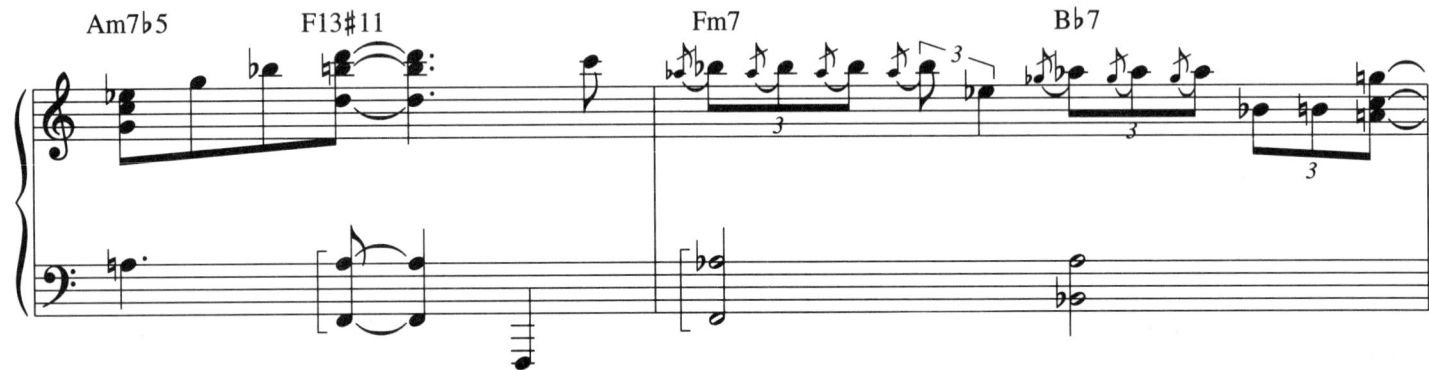
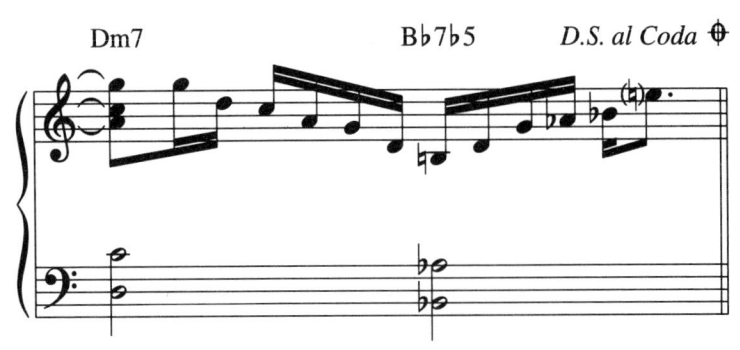
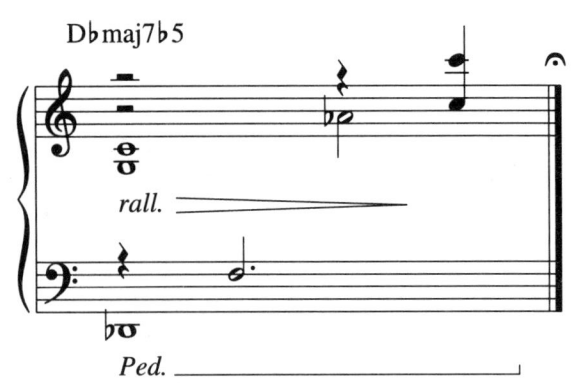

Two Bass Hit

by Dizzy Gillespie and John Lewis

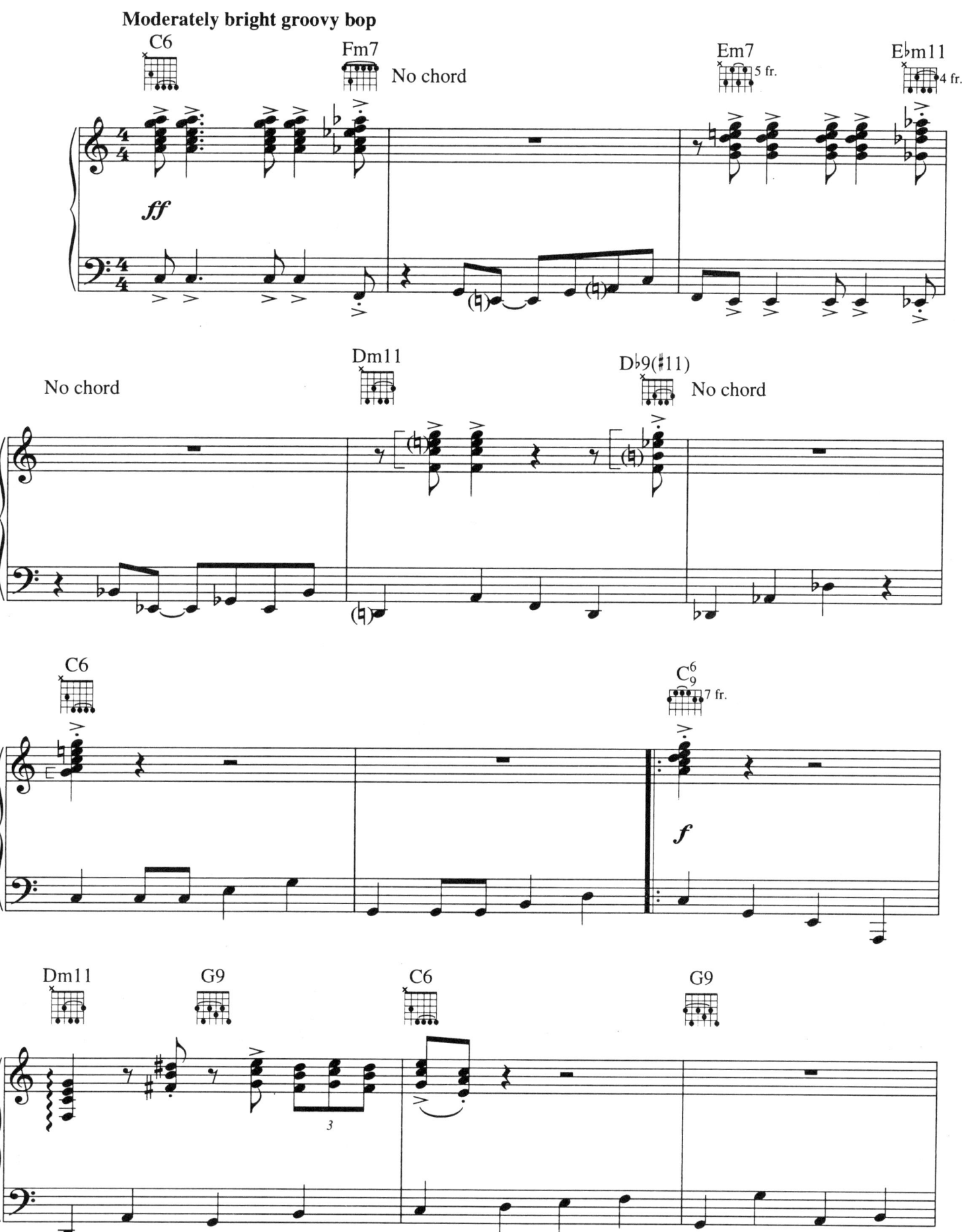

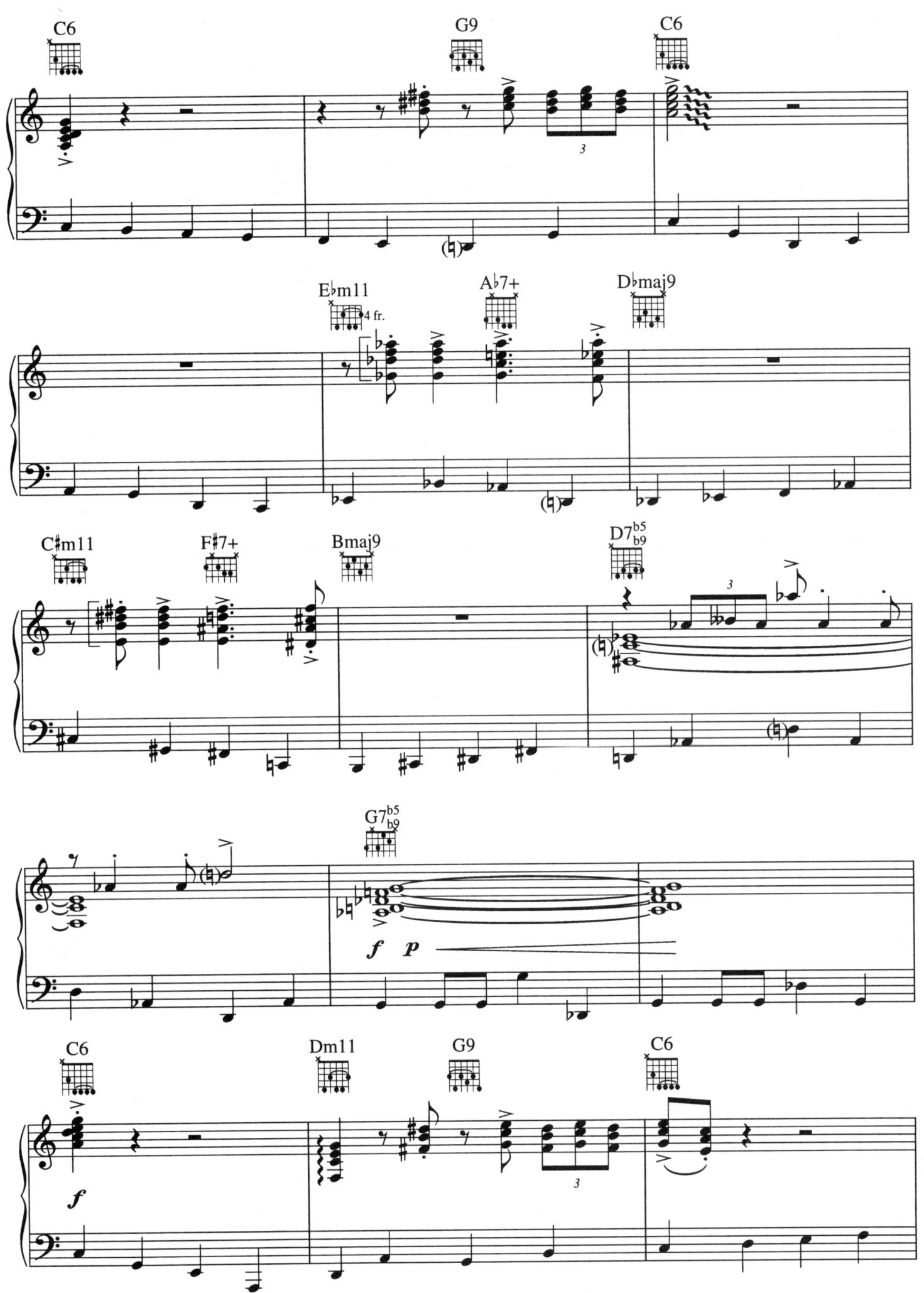

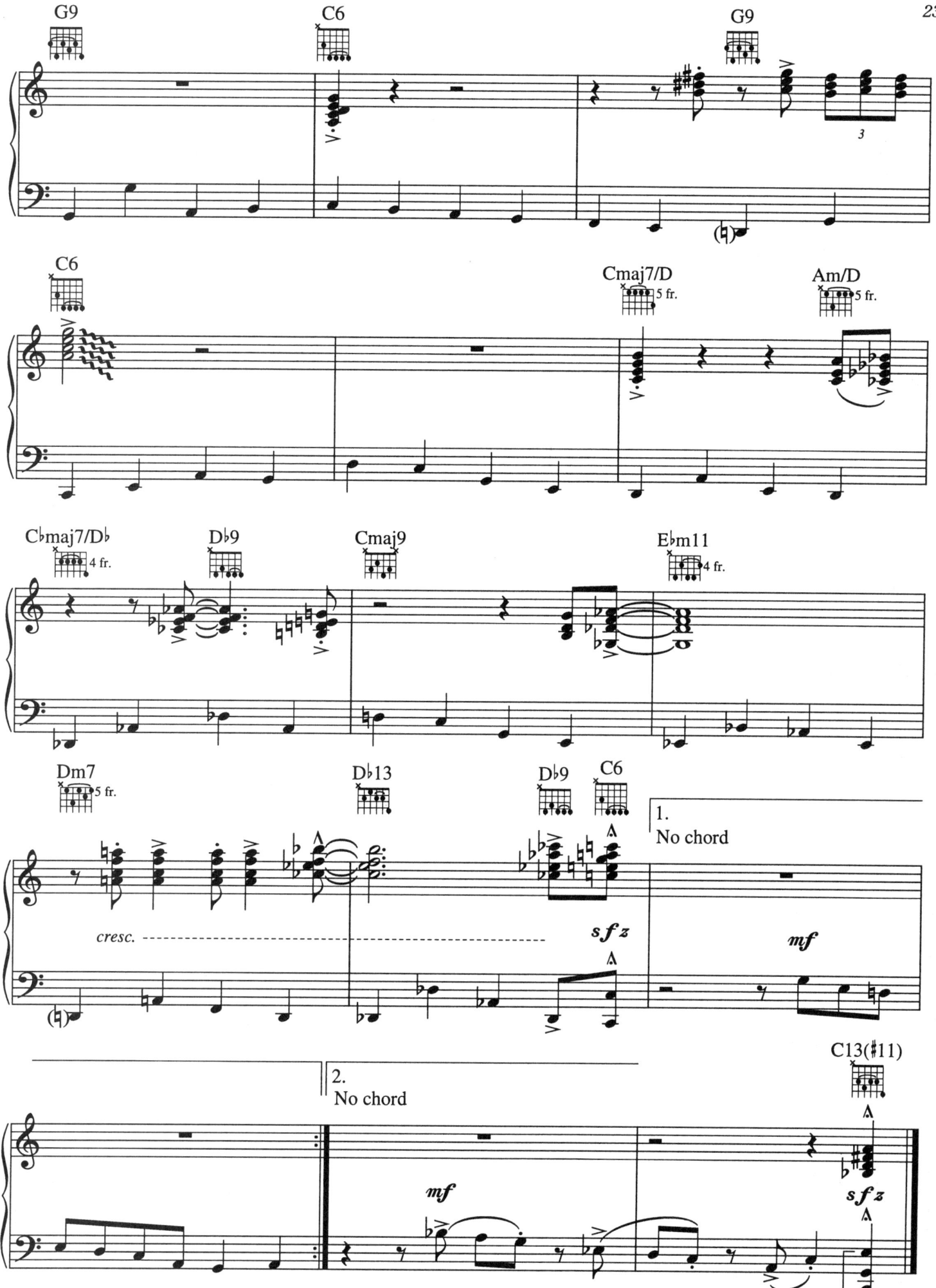

Soul Sauce
(a/k/a Guachi Guaro)
by Dizzie Gillespie and Chano Pozo

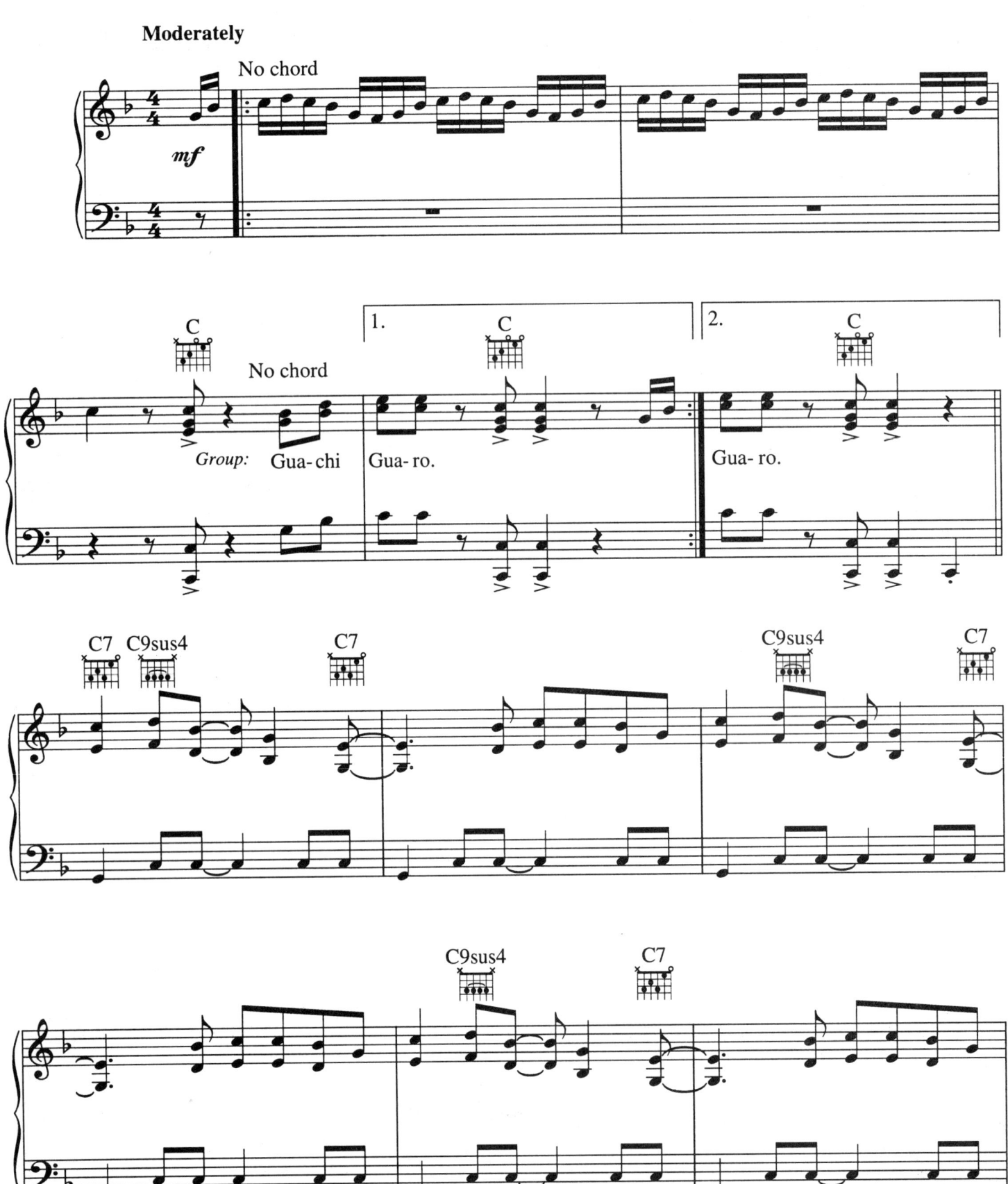

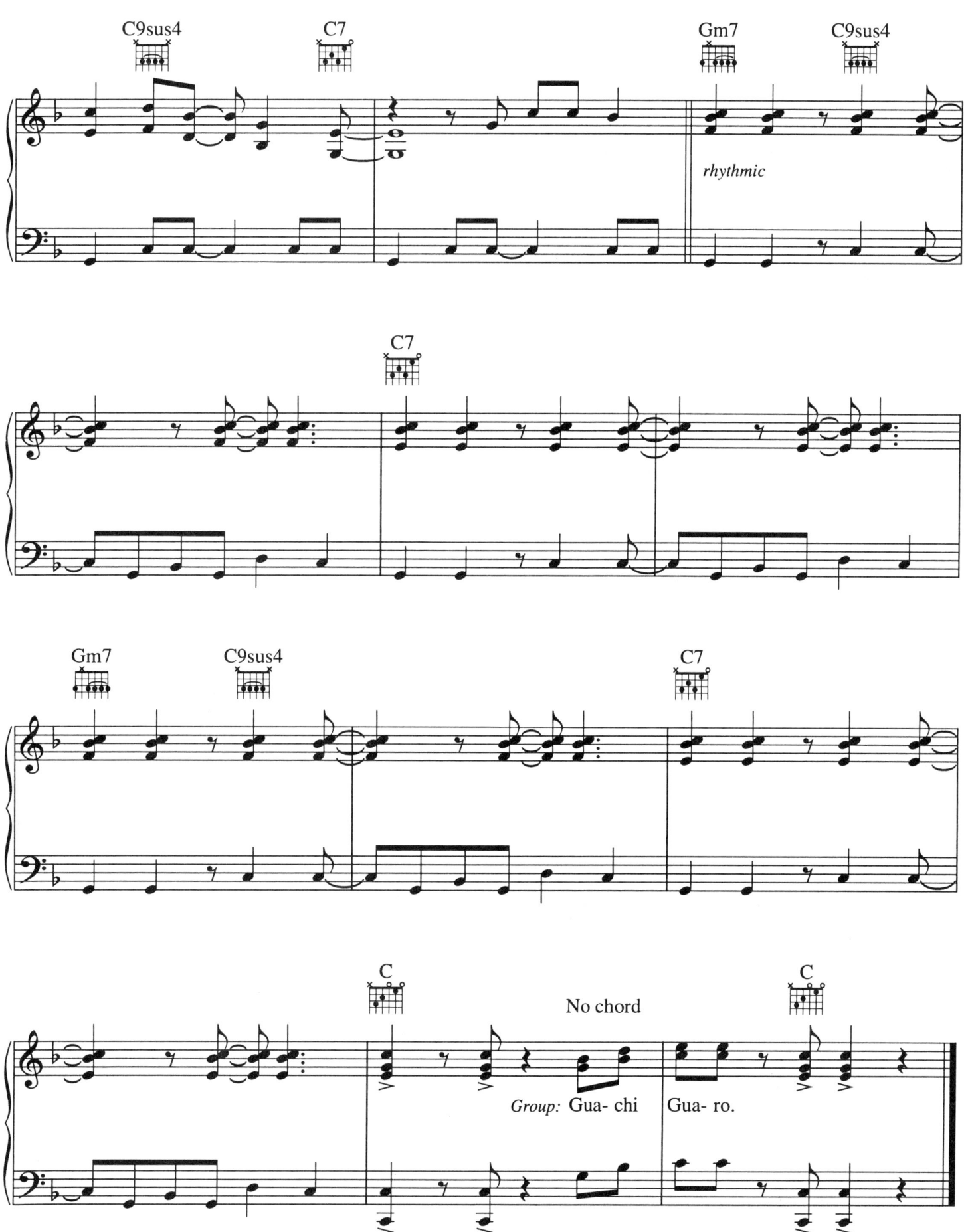

Allen's Alley

by Denzil Best

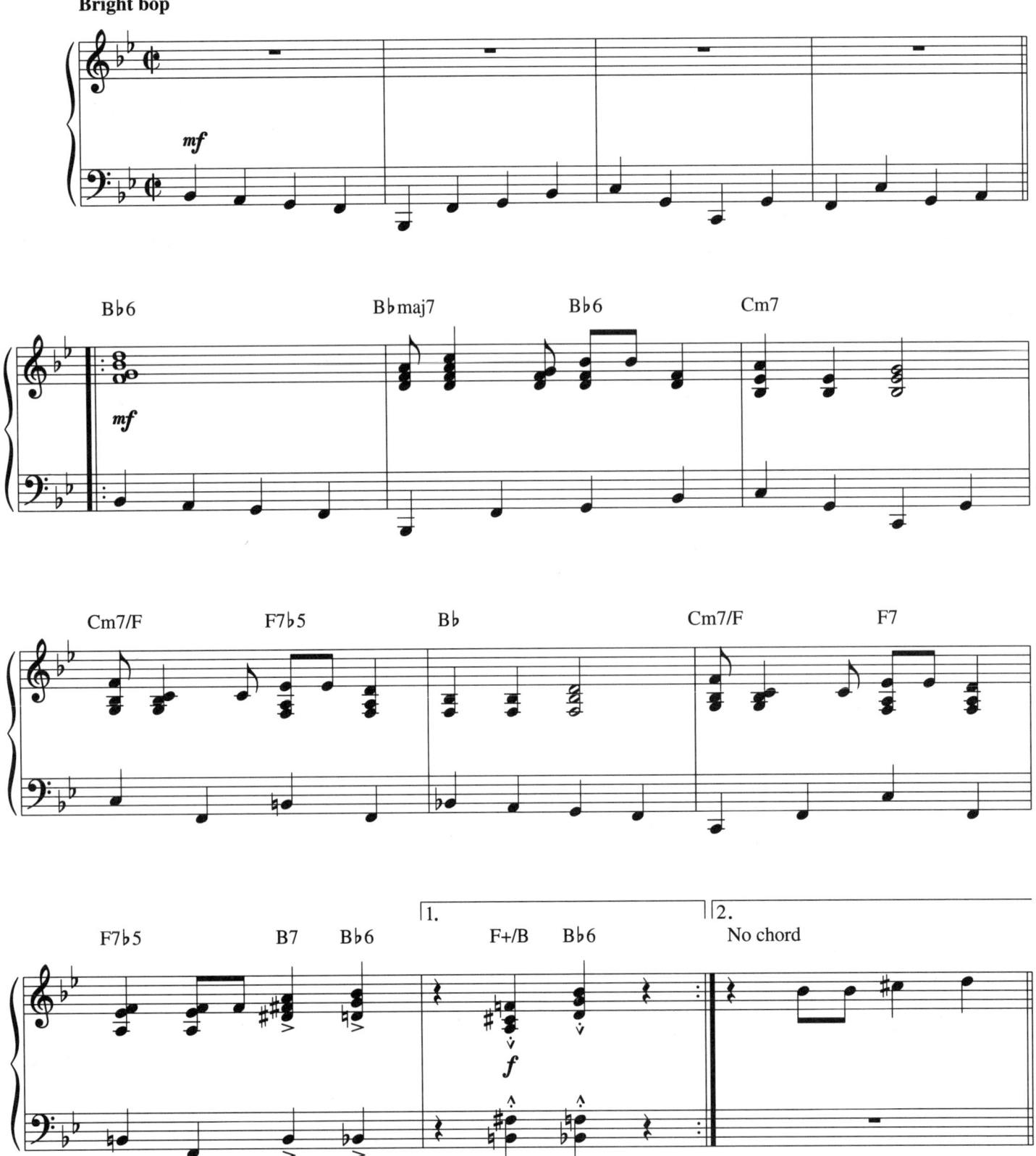

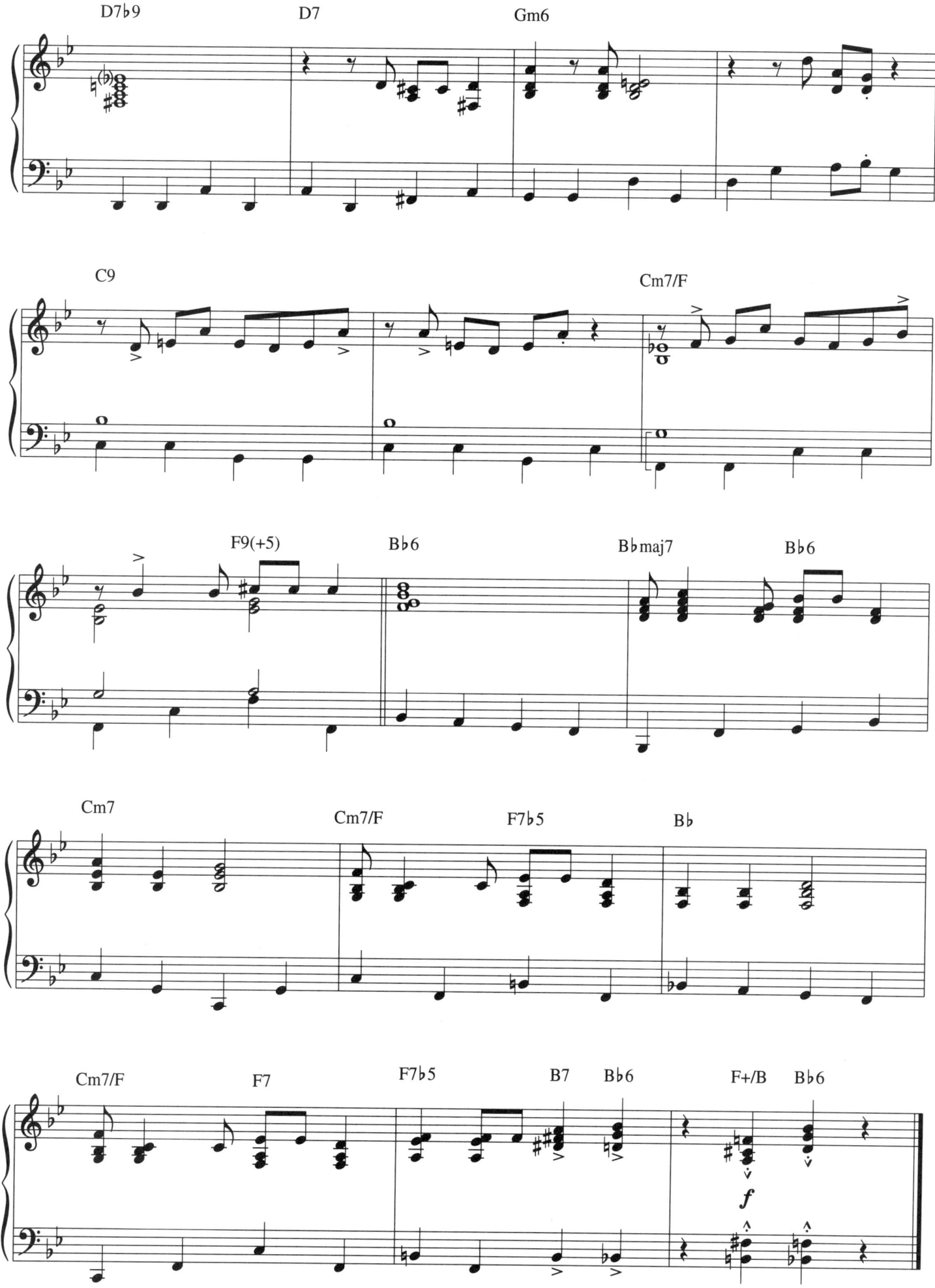

Bouncin' With Bud

by Earl 'Bud' Powell and Walter 'Gil' Fuller

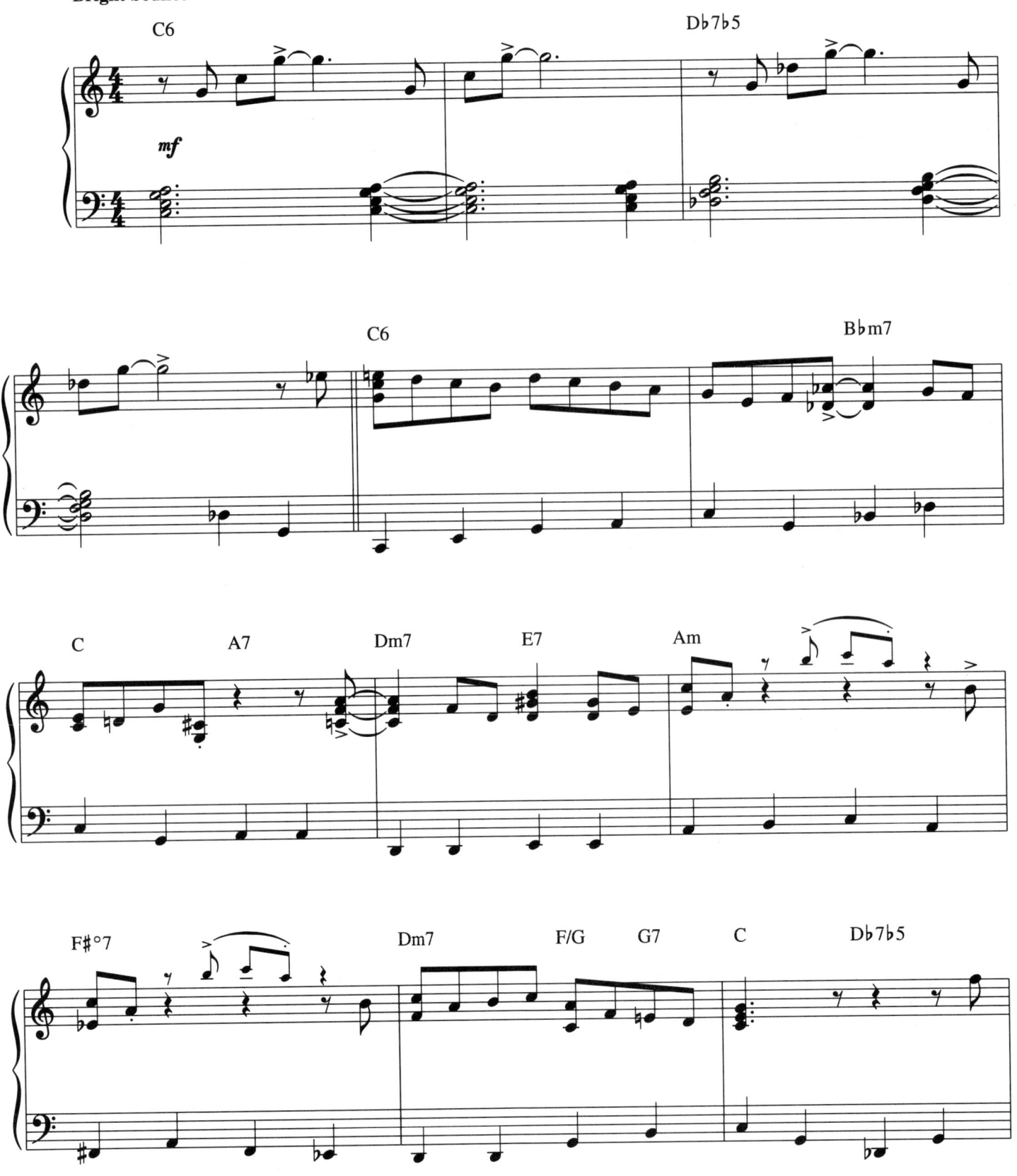

Copyright © 1947 (Renewed) by Embassy Music Corporation (BMI) and Music Sales Corporation (ASCAP)
All rights outside the United States controlled by Music Sales Corporation
International Copyright Secured. All Rights Reserved.

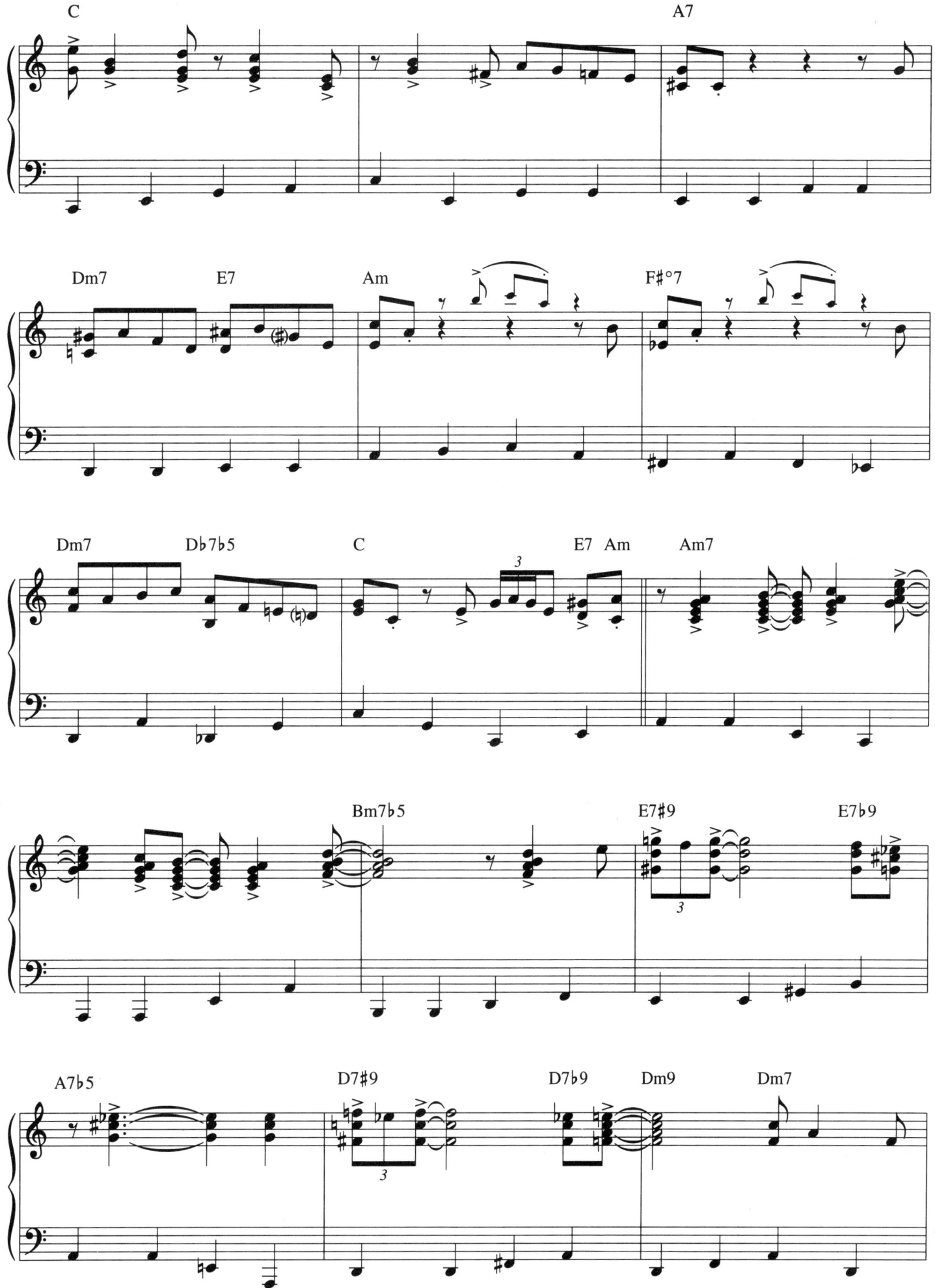

Db9b5 Db7b5
C6
Bbm7
C A7
Dm7 E7
Am
F#°7
Dm7 F/G G7
C
G#°7 Am
E7 Am
C#°7 Dm
A7 Dm Ab9 G9
Db7 C6
dim.
p

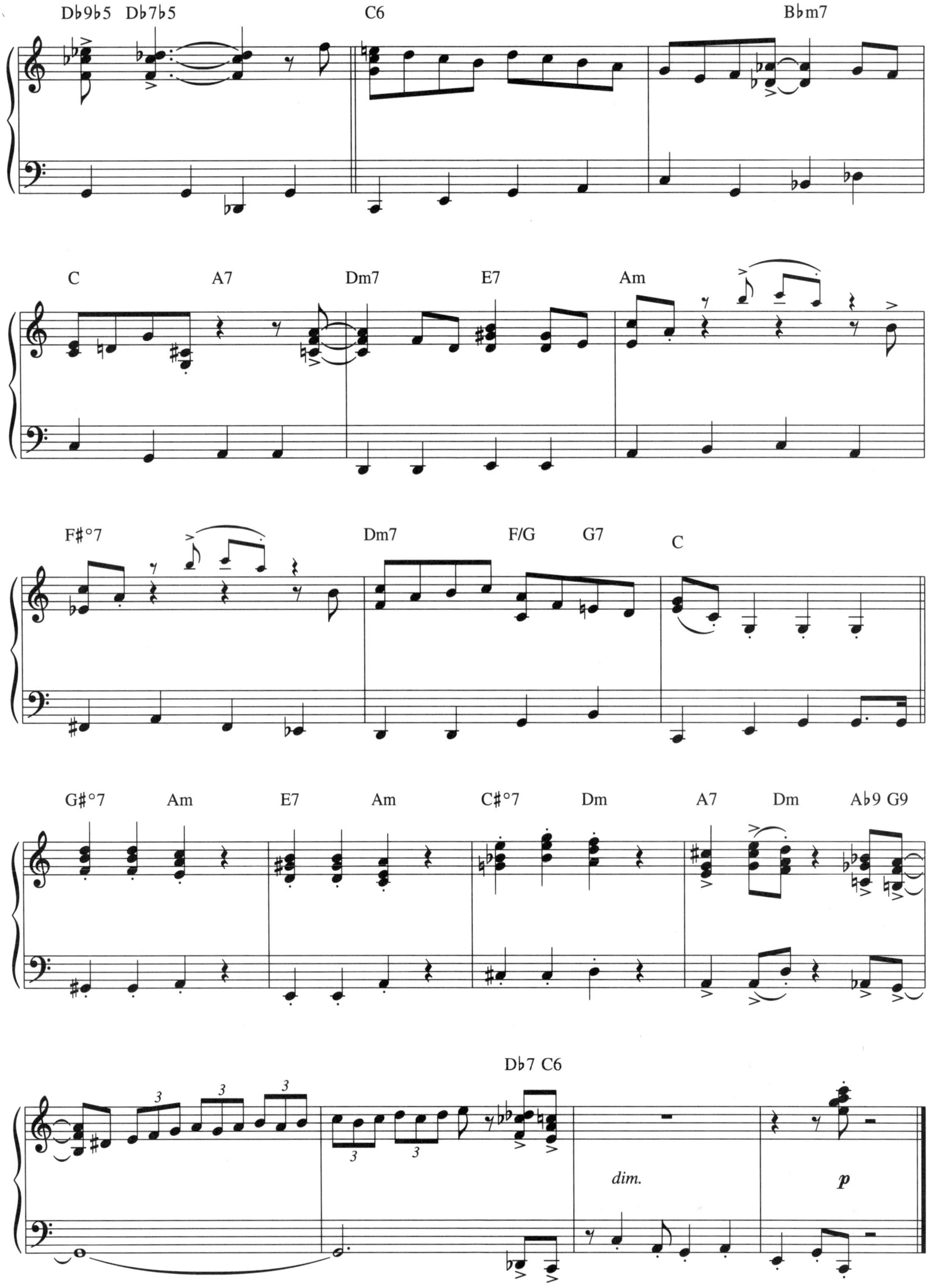

Epistrophy

by Thelonious Monk and Kenny Clark

Medium bop

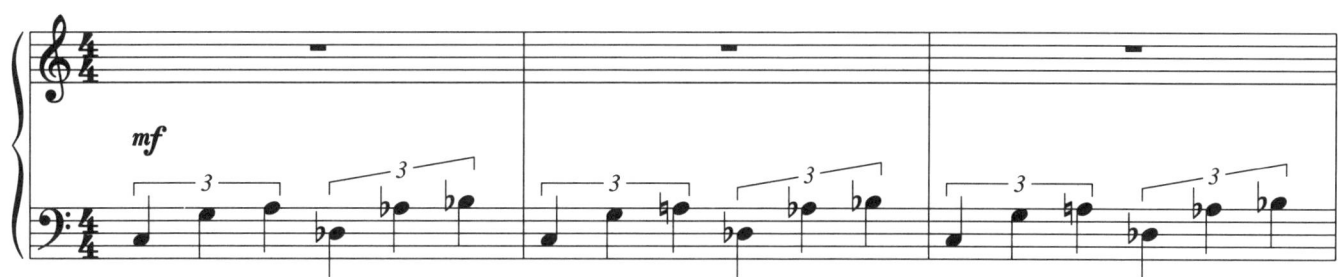
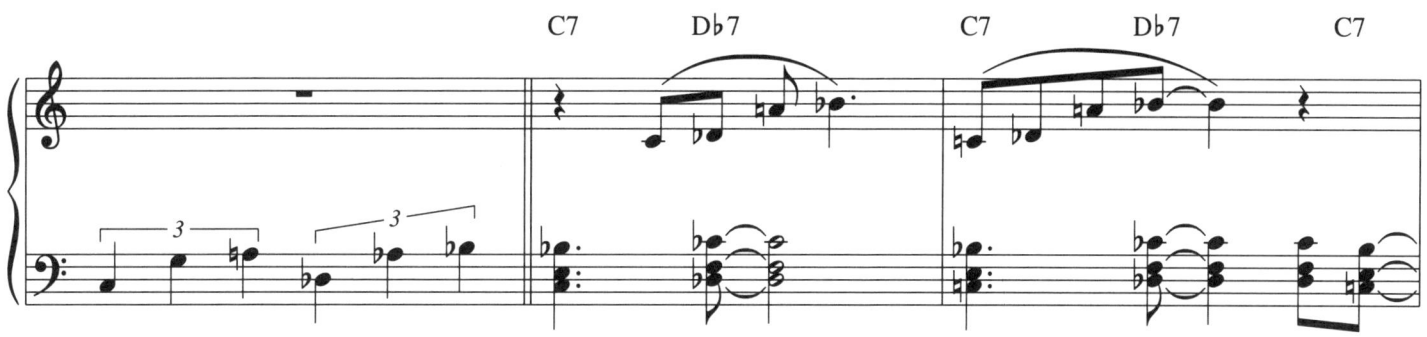
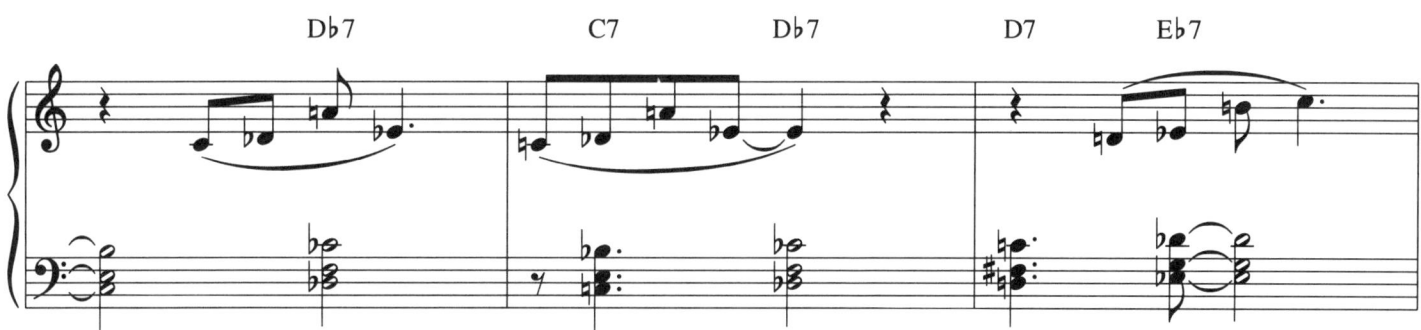
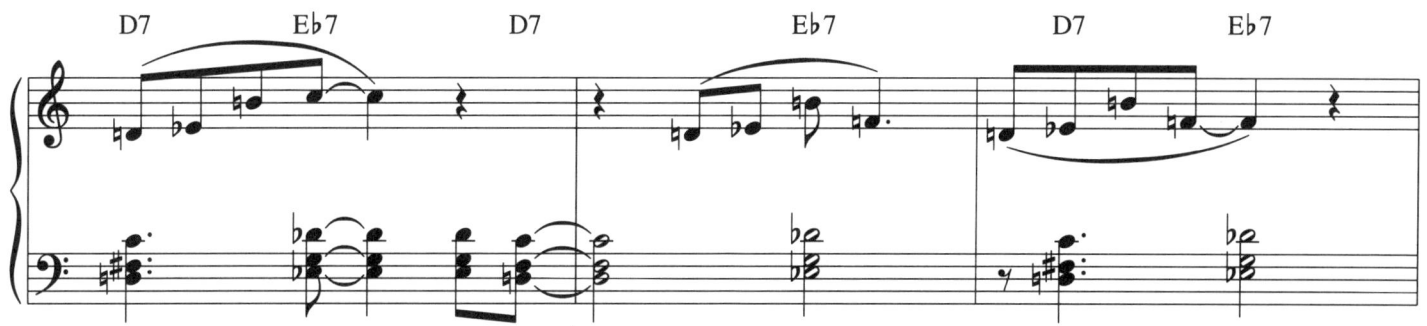

Copyright © 1947 (Renewed) by Embassy Music Corporation (BMI) and Music Sales Corporation (ASCAP)
All rights outside the United States controlled by Music Sales Corporation
International Copyright Secured. All Rights Reserved.

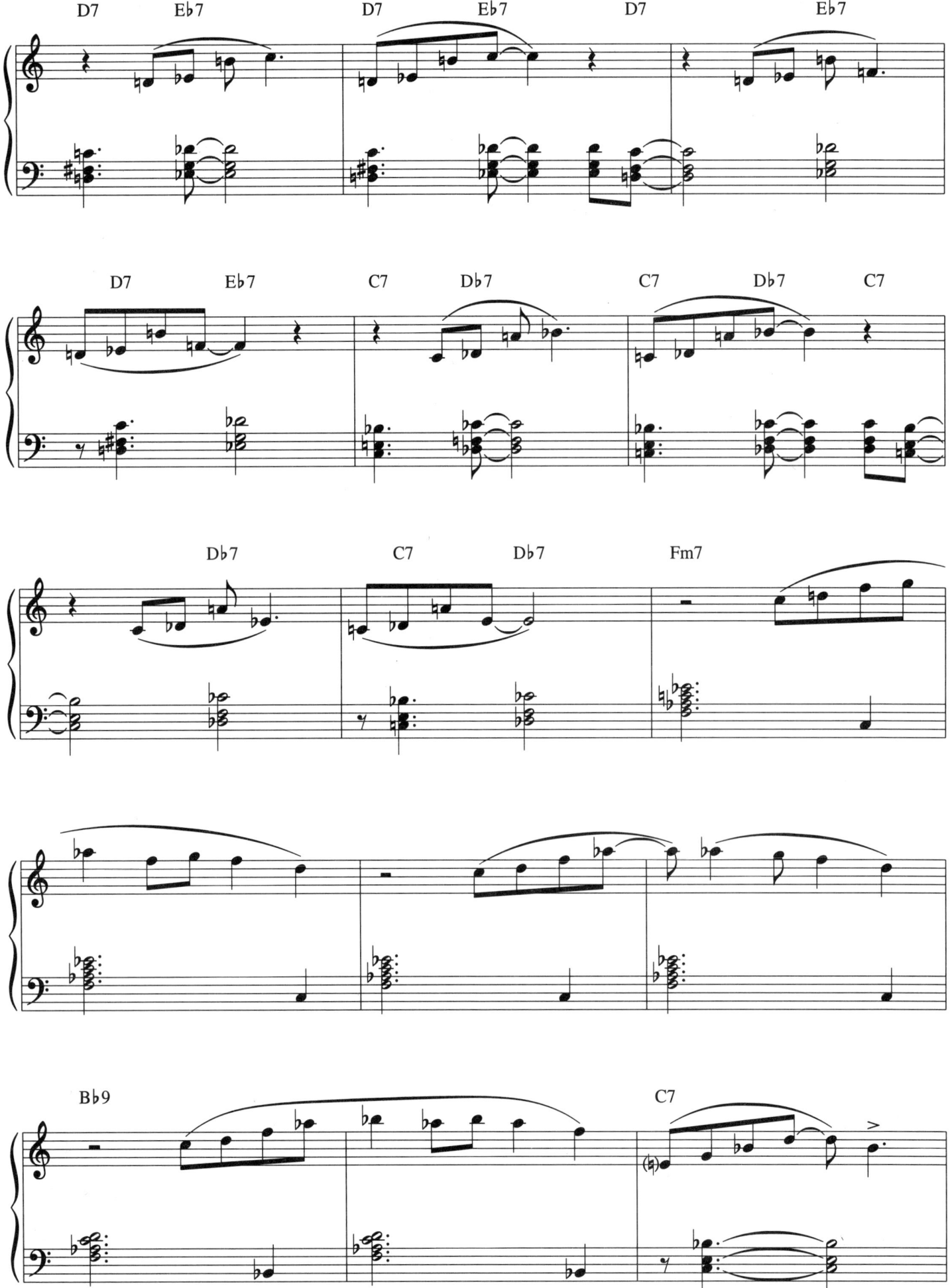

Db7
D7
Eb7
D7
Eb7
D7
Eb7
D7
Eb7
C7
Db7
C7
Db7
C7
Db7
C7
Db7
G7
Abm9
Cmaj7
No Chord
mf
rall.
C7#9
p

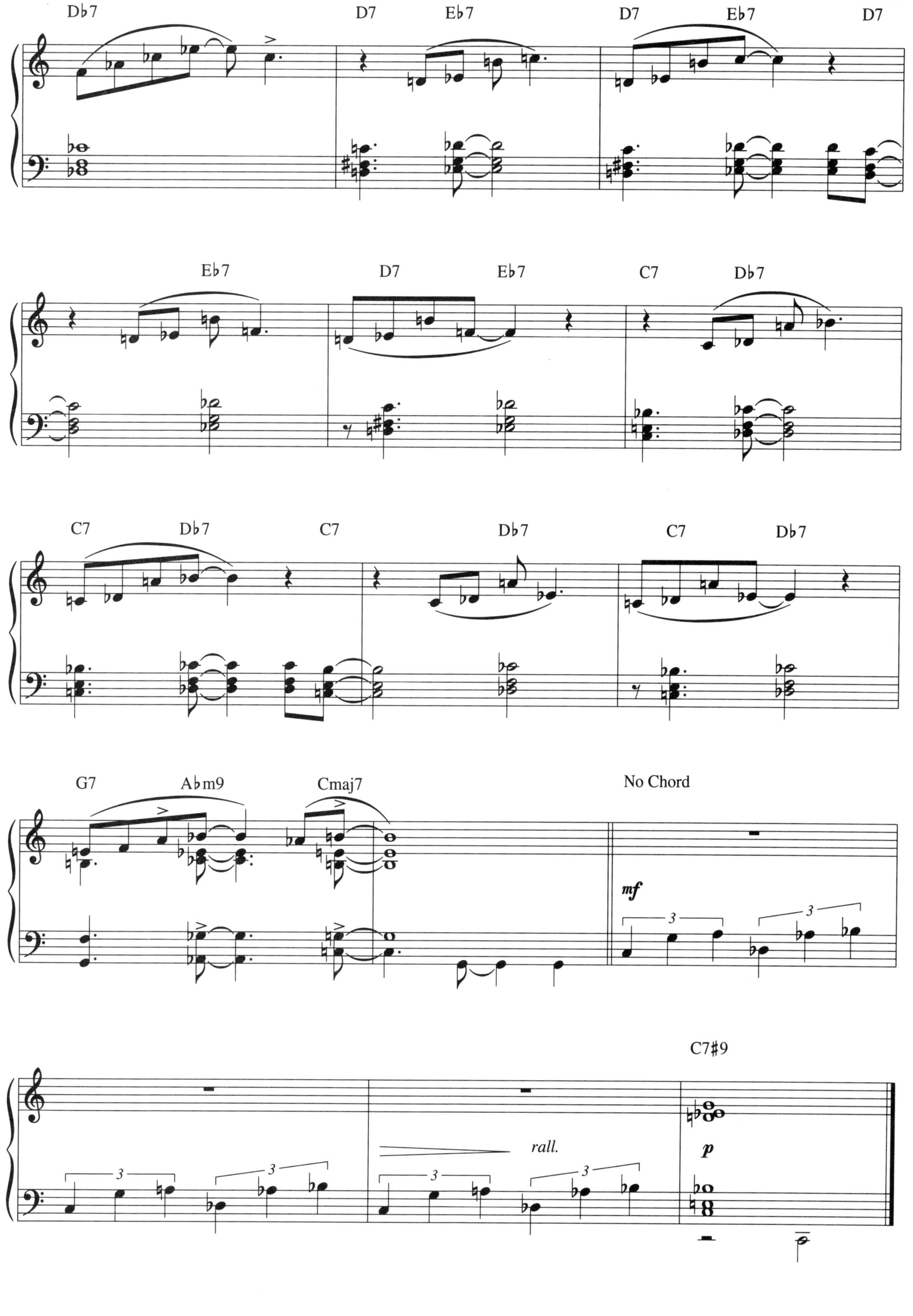

Ladybird
by Tadd Dameron

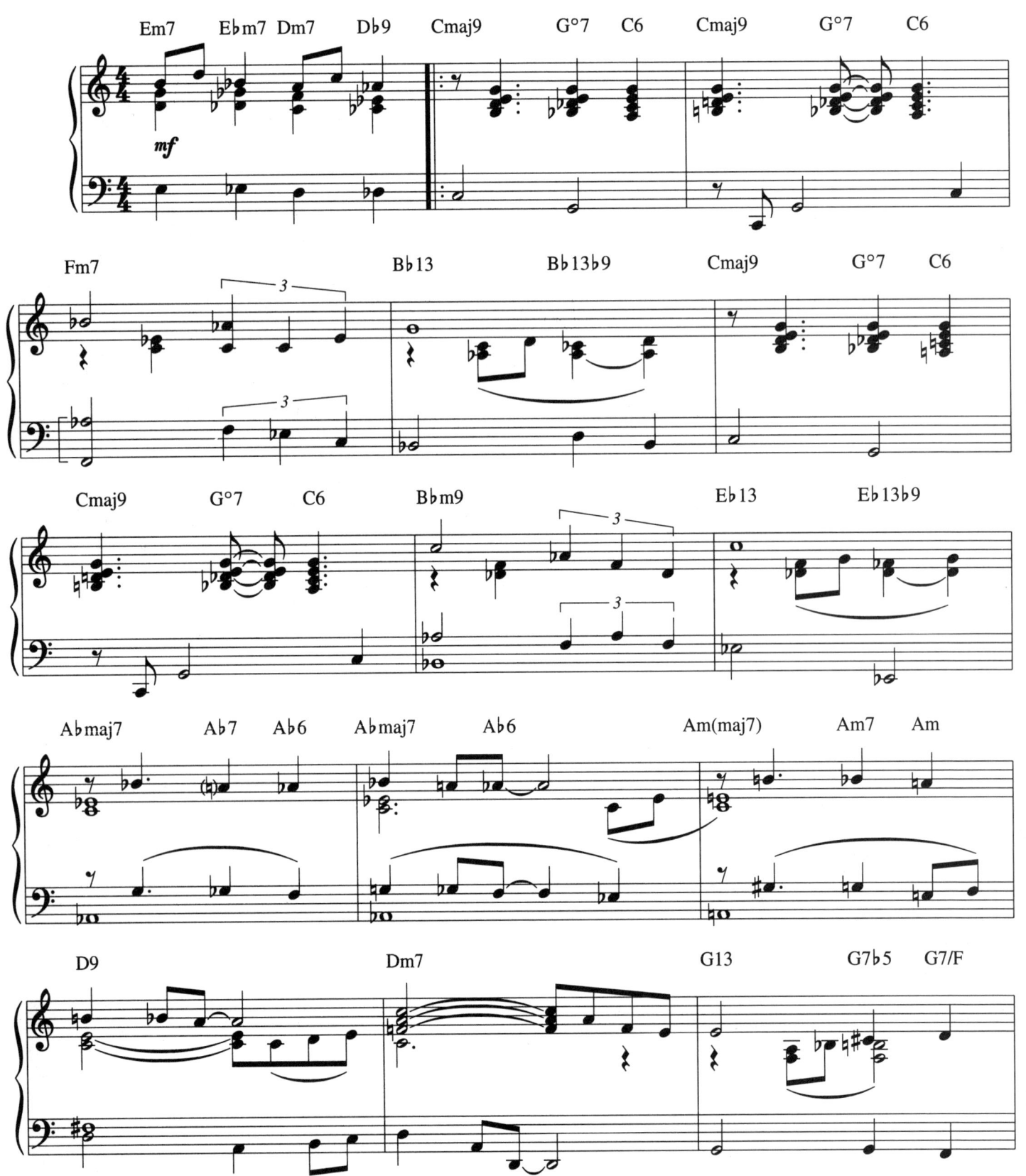

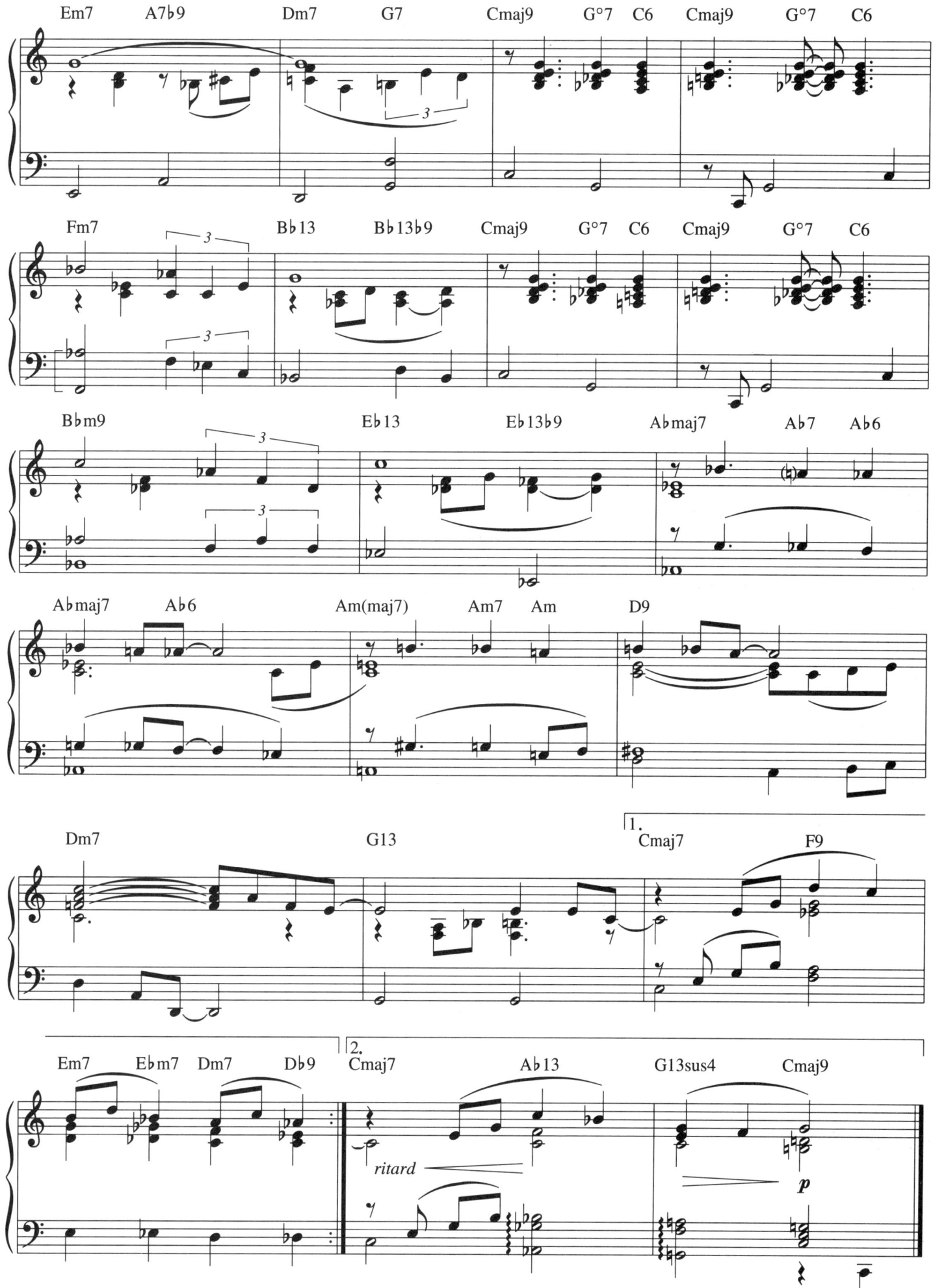

Manteca

by John 'Dizzy' Gillespie, Walter G. Fuller and Luciano Pozo Gonzales

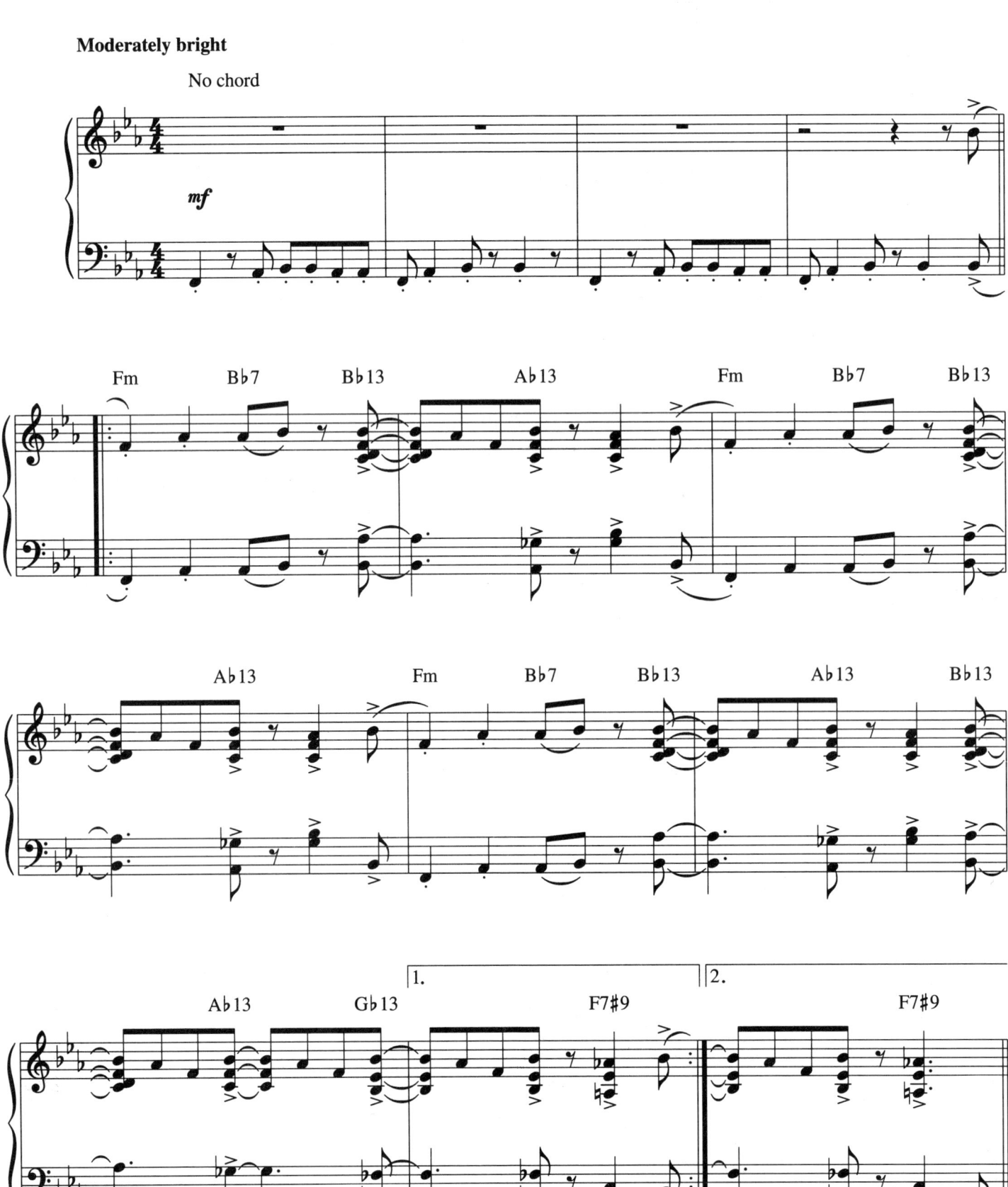

Copyright © 1948 (Renewed) by Music Sales Corporation (ASCAP) and EMI Music Publishing
All rights outside of the United States controlled by Music Sales Corporation
International Copyright Secured. All Rights Reserved.

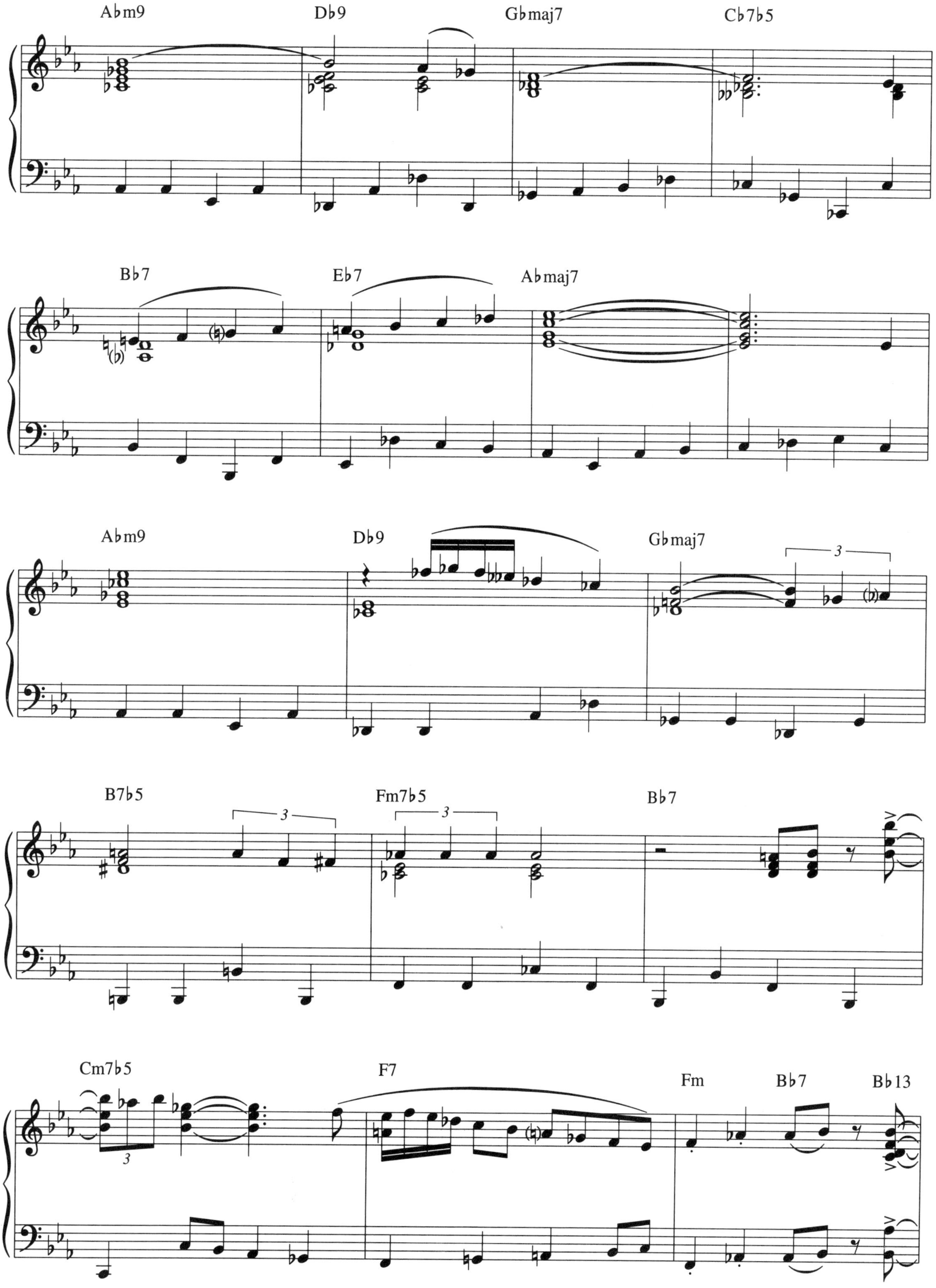
Abm9
Db9
Gbmaj7
Cb7b5
Bb7
Eb7
Abmaj7
Abm9
Db9
Gbmaj7
3
B7b5
3
Fm7b5
3
Bb7
Cm7b5
3
F7
Fm
Bb7
Bb13

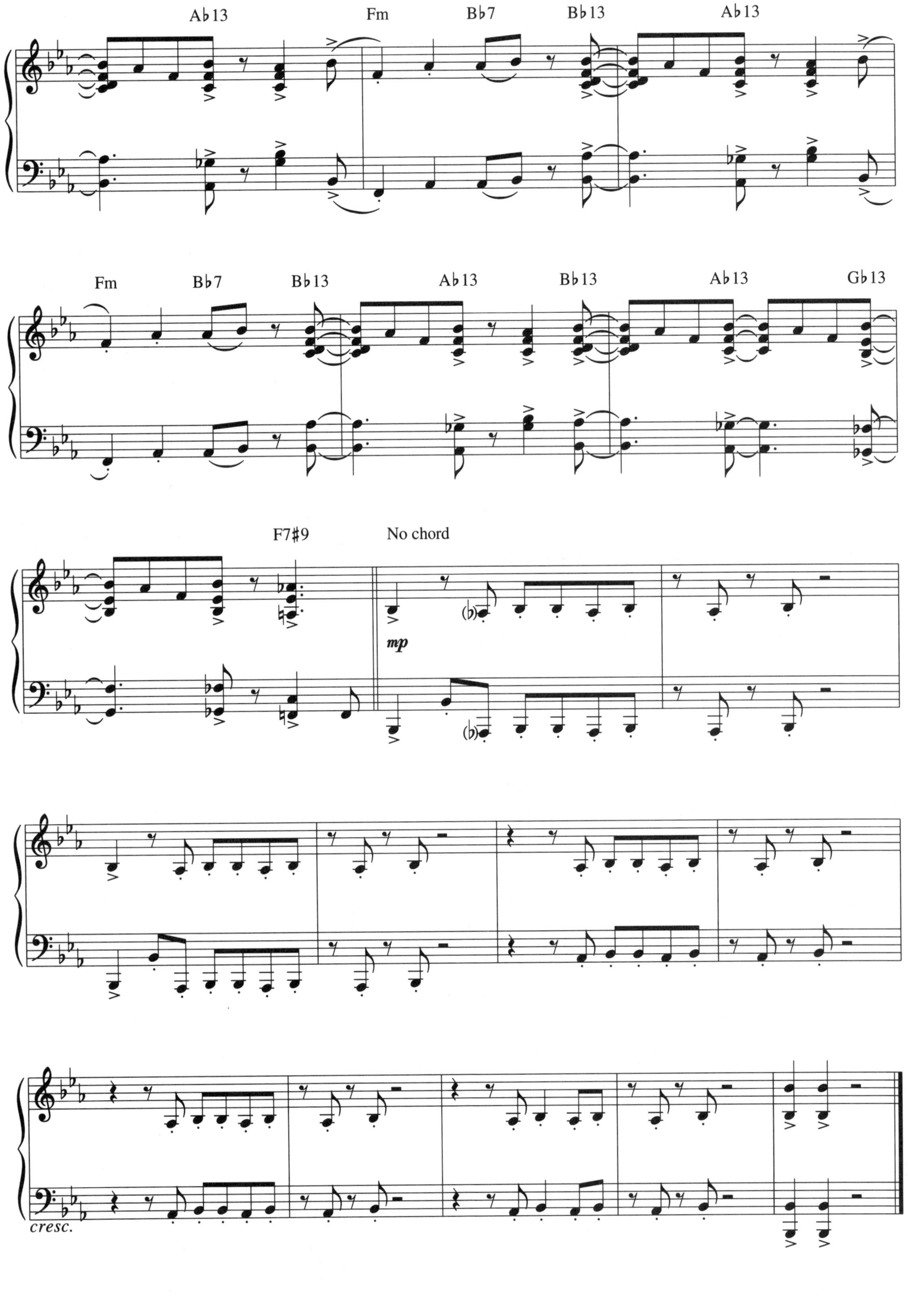
Ab13
Fm
Bb7
Bb13
Ab13
Fm
Bb7
Bb13
Ab13
Bb13
Ab13
Gb13
F7#9
No chord
mp
cresc.

Thelonious

by Thelonious Monk

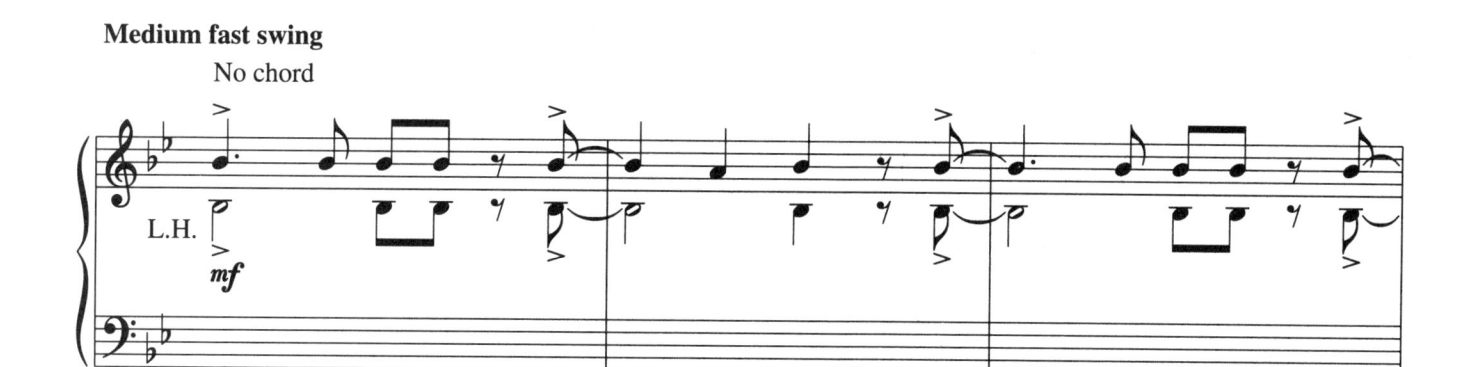

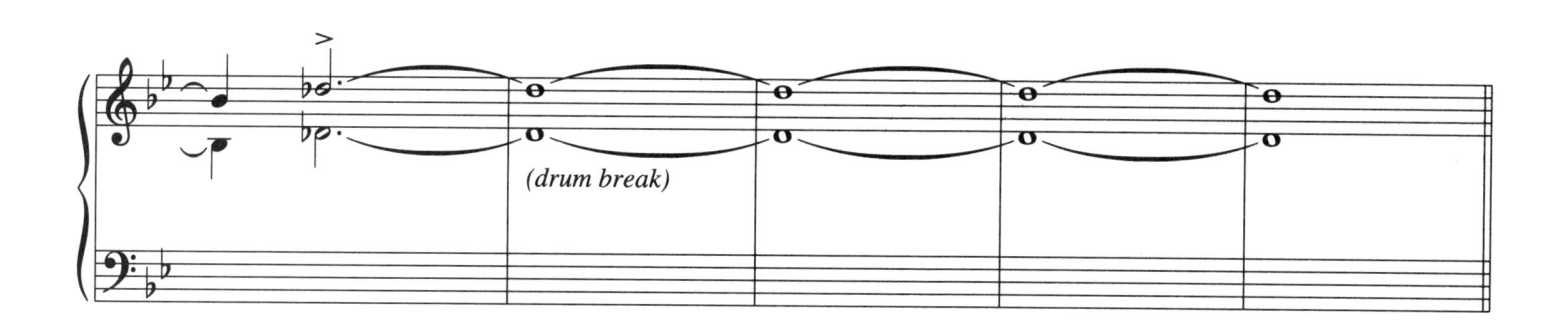

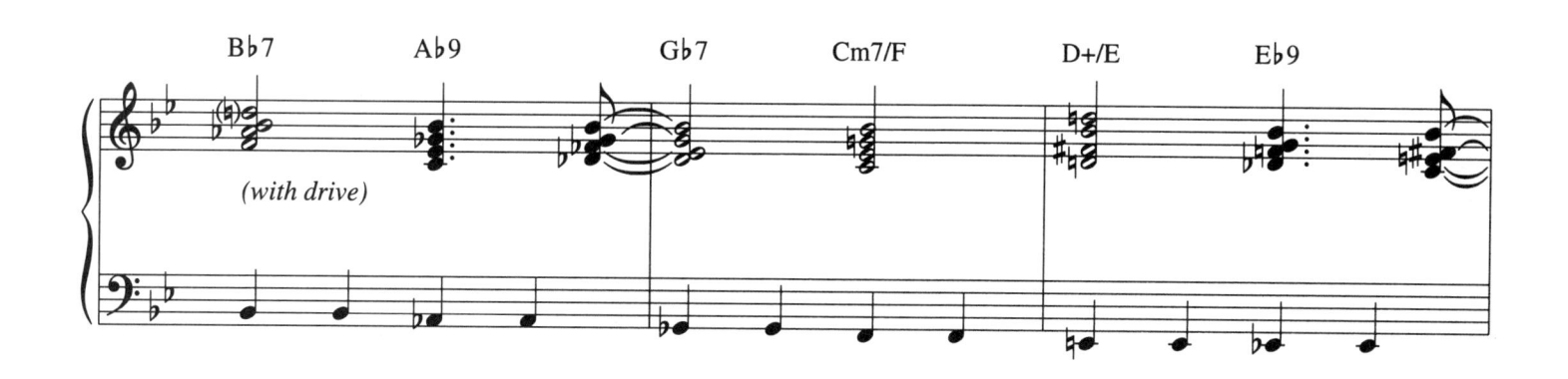

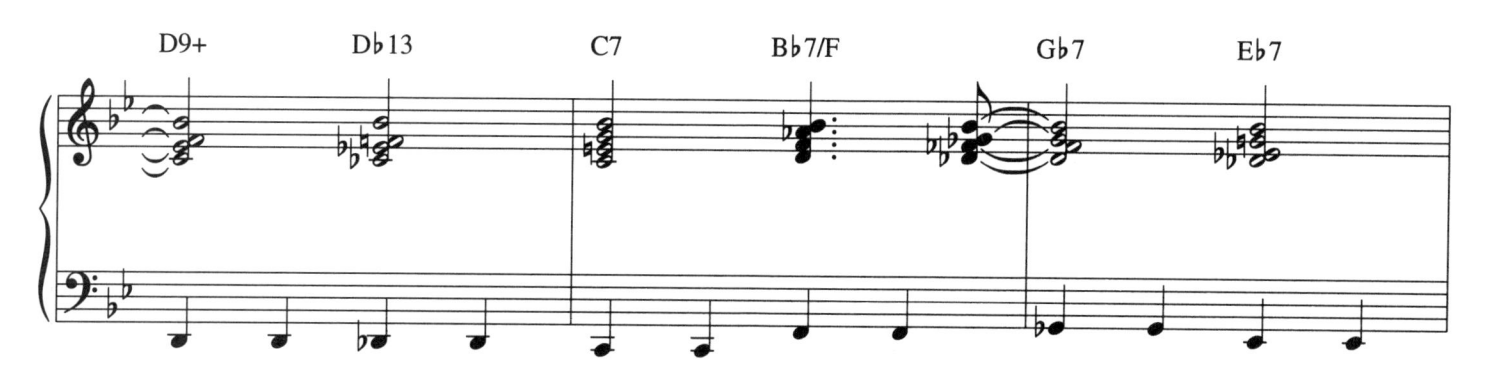

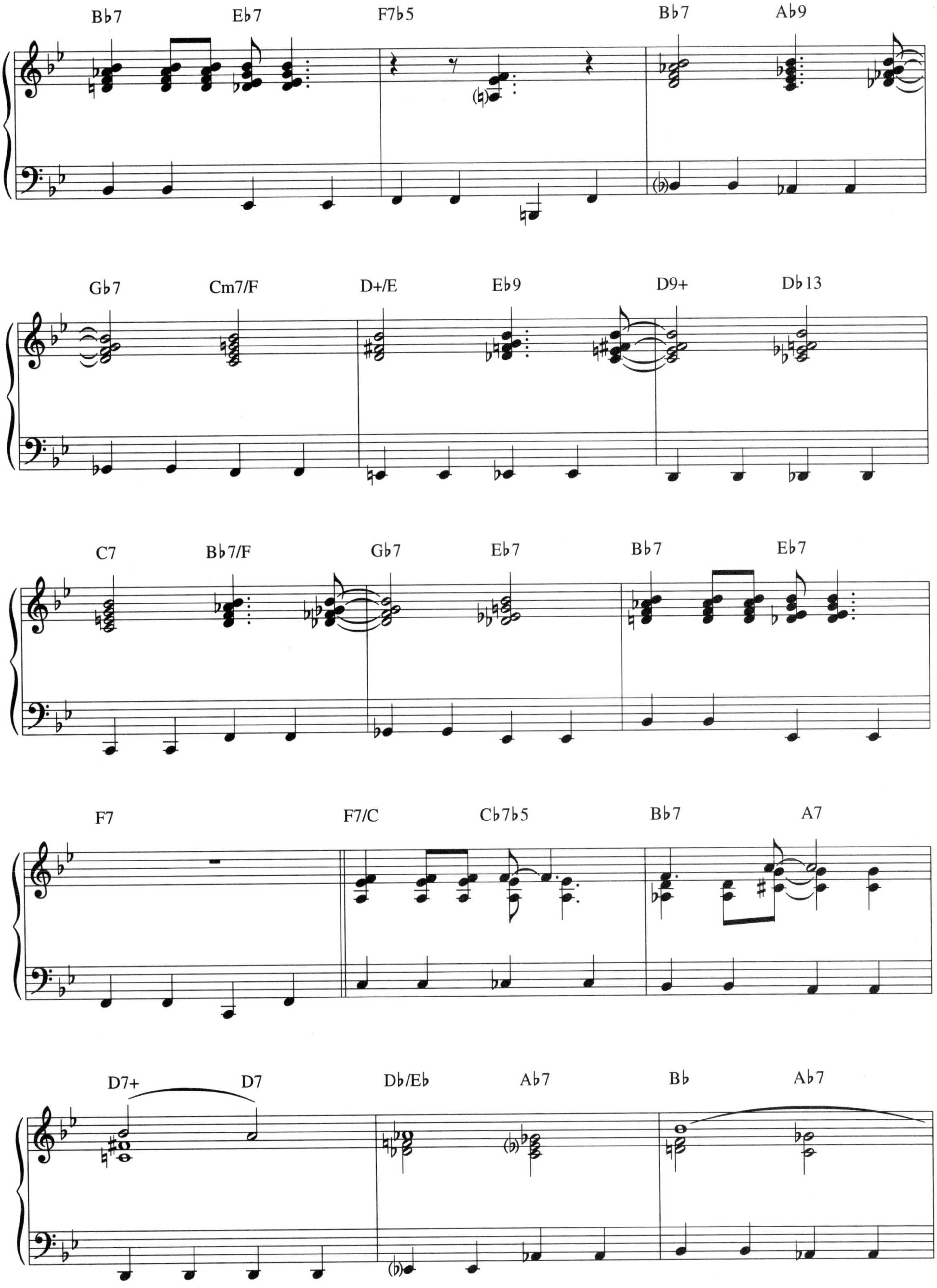
Bb7 Eb7 F7b5 Bb7 Ab9
Gb7 Cm7/F D+/E Eb9 D9+ Db13
C7 Bb7/F Gb7 Eb7 Bb7 Eb7
F7 F7/C Cb7b5 Bb7 A7
D7+ D7 Db/Eb Ab7 Bb Ab7

41

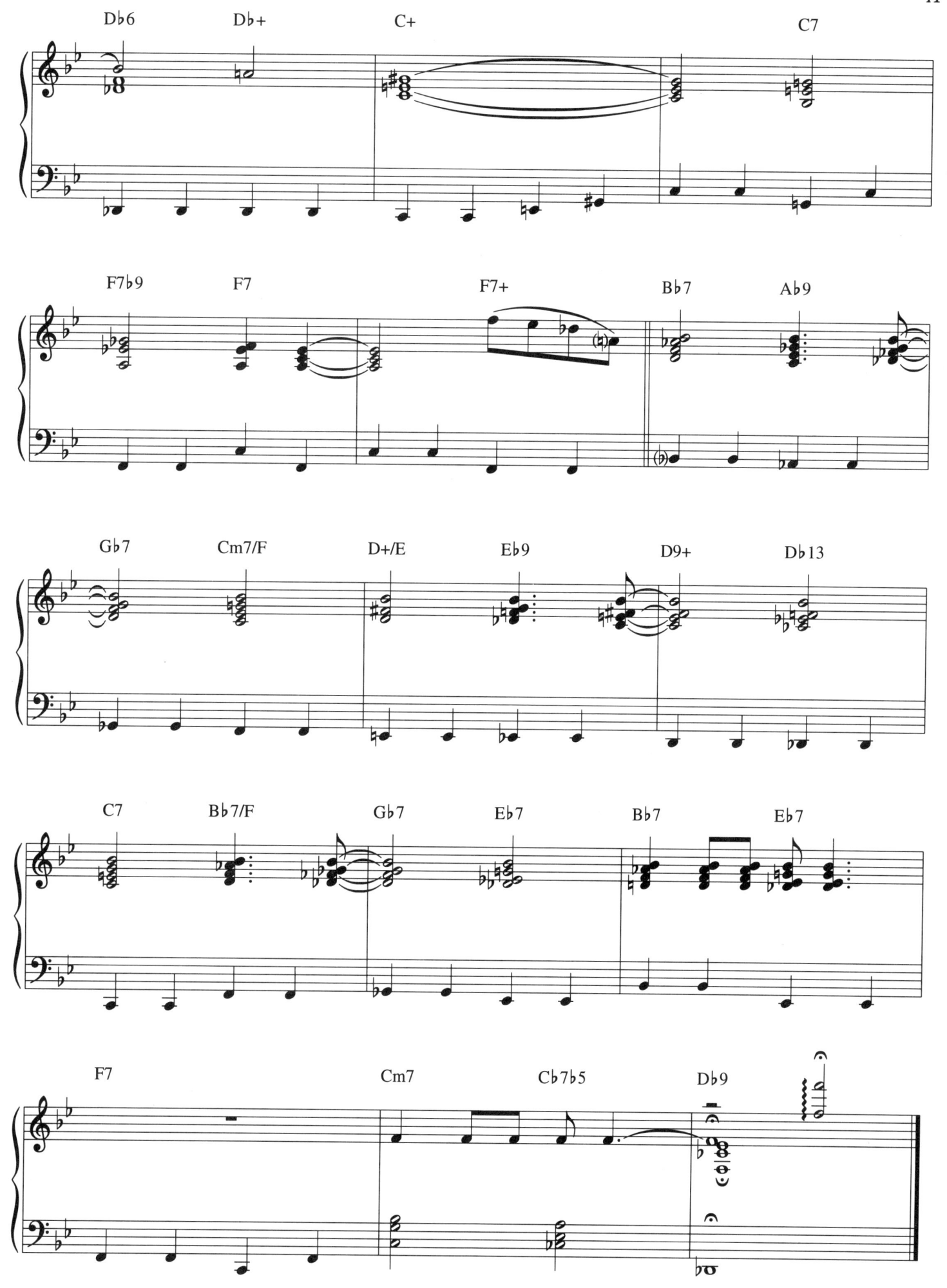

Wouldn't You
(a/k/a Woodyn't You)
by Dizzy Gillespie

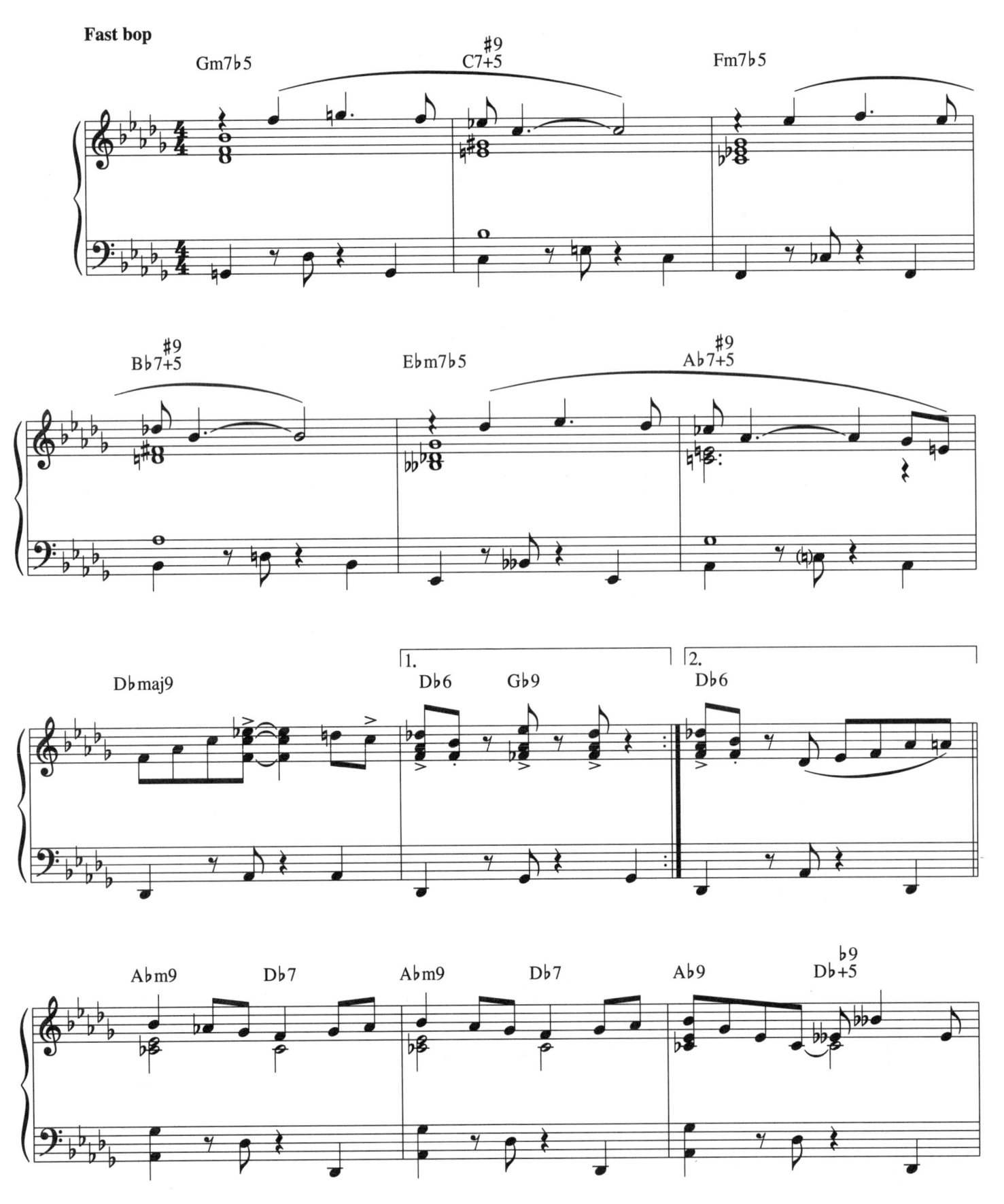

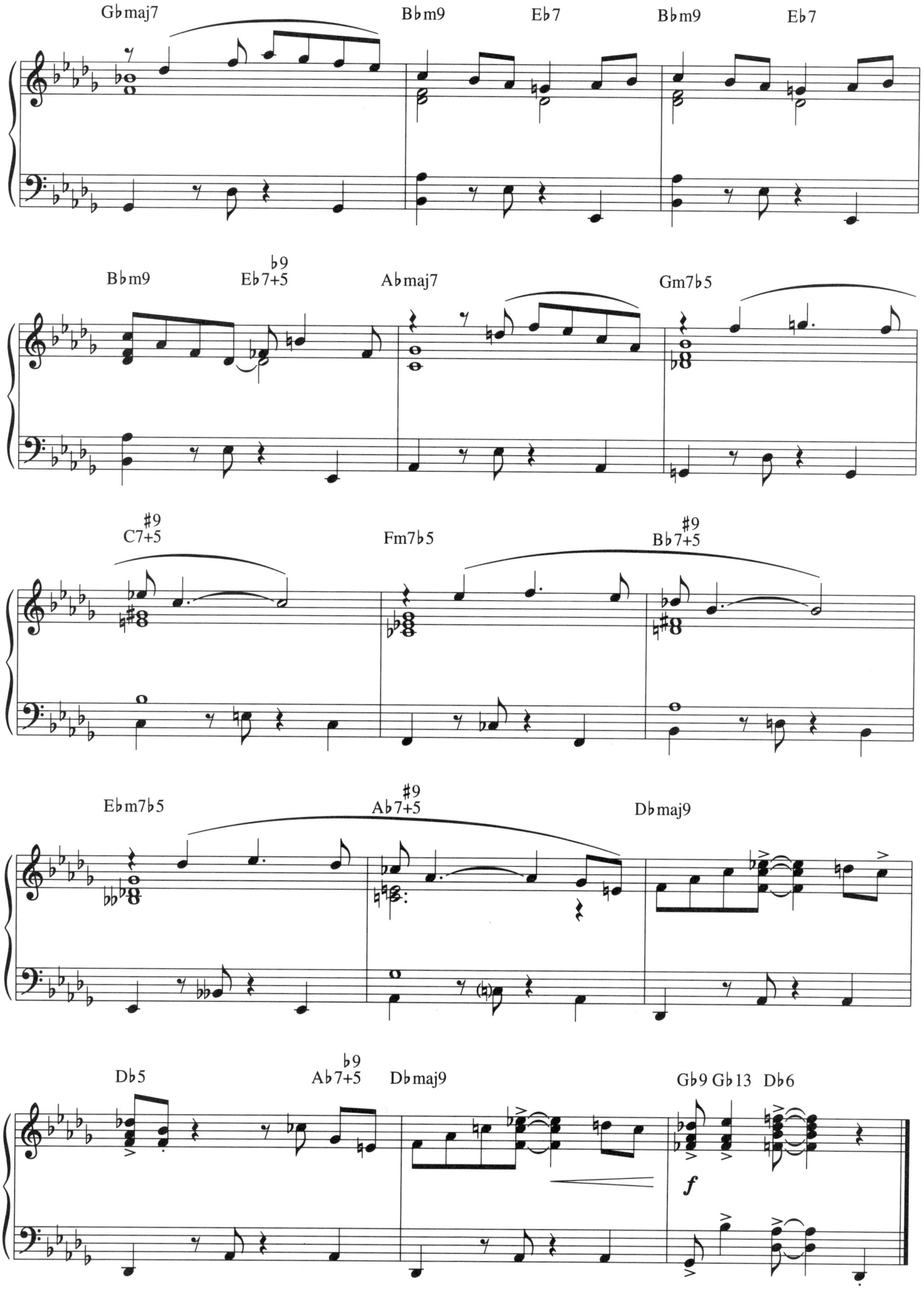
Gb maj7
Bb m9
Eb7
Bb m9
Eb7
Bb m9
b9 Eb7+5
Ab maj7
Gm7b5
#9 C7+5
Fm7b5
#9 Bb7+5
Ebm7b5
#9 Ab7+5
Db maj9
Db5
b9 Ab7+5
Db maj9
Gb9
Gb13
Db6
f

Off Minor
(a/k/a What Now)
by Thelonious Monk

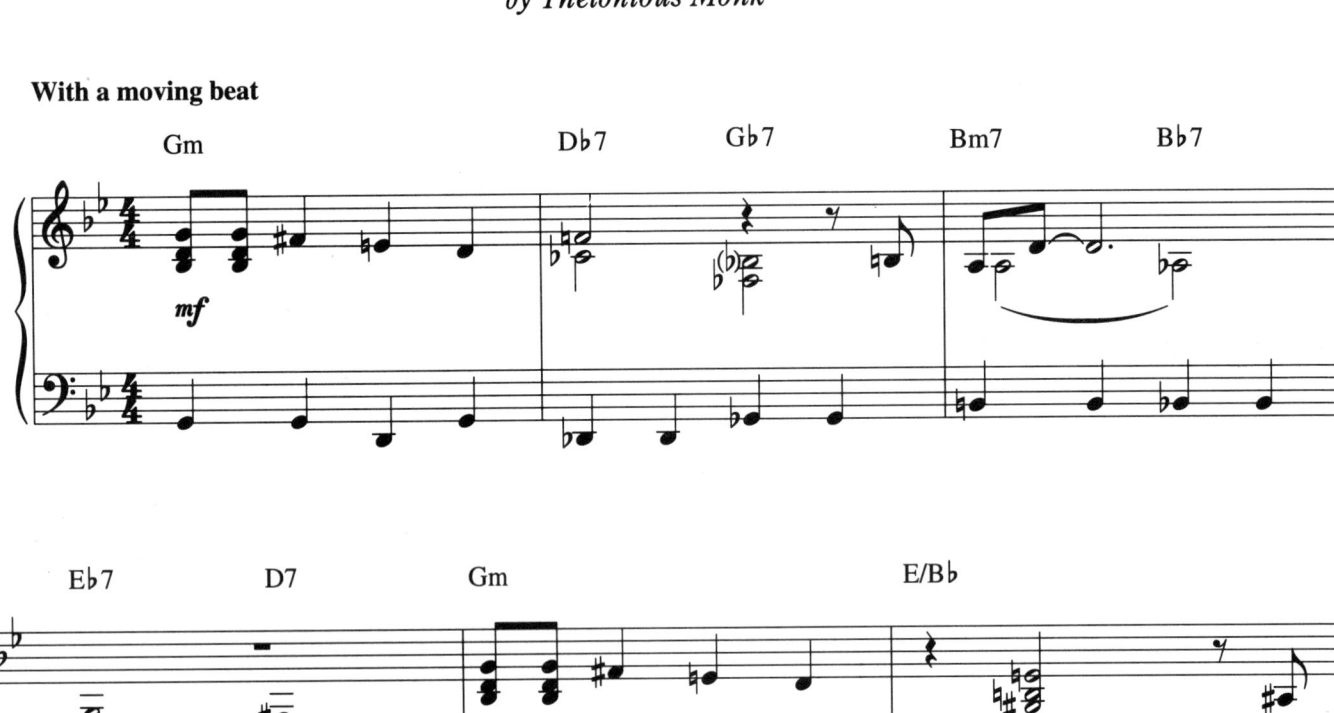

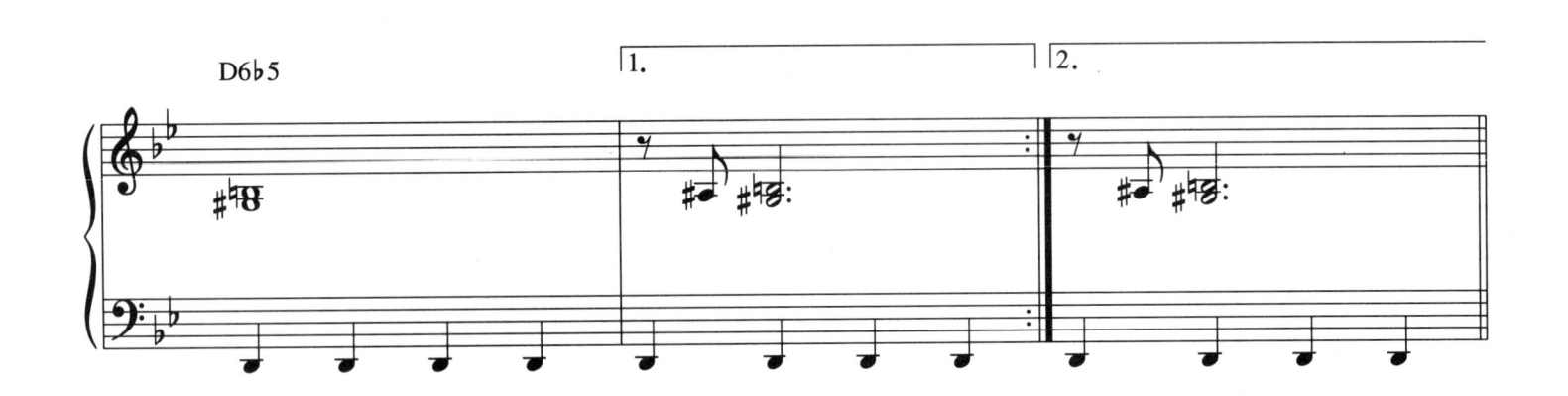

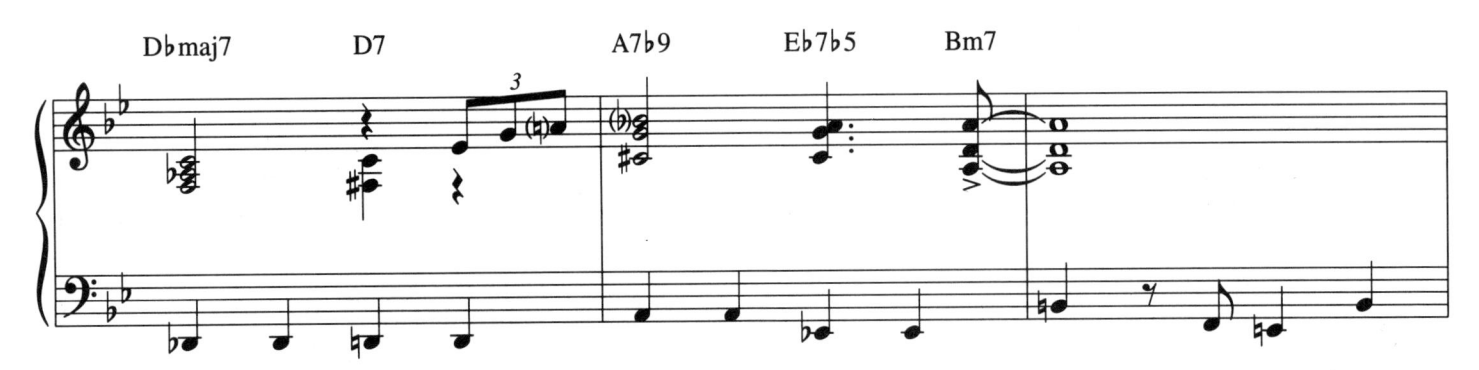

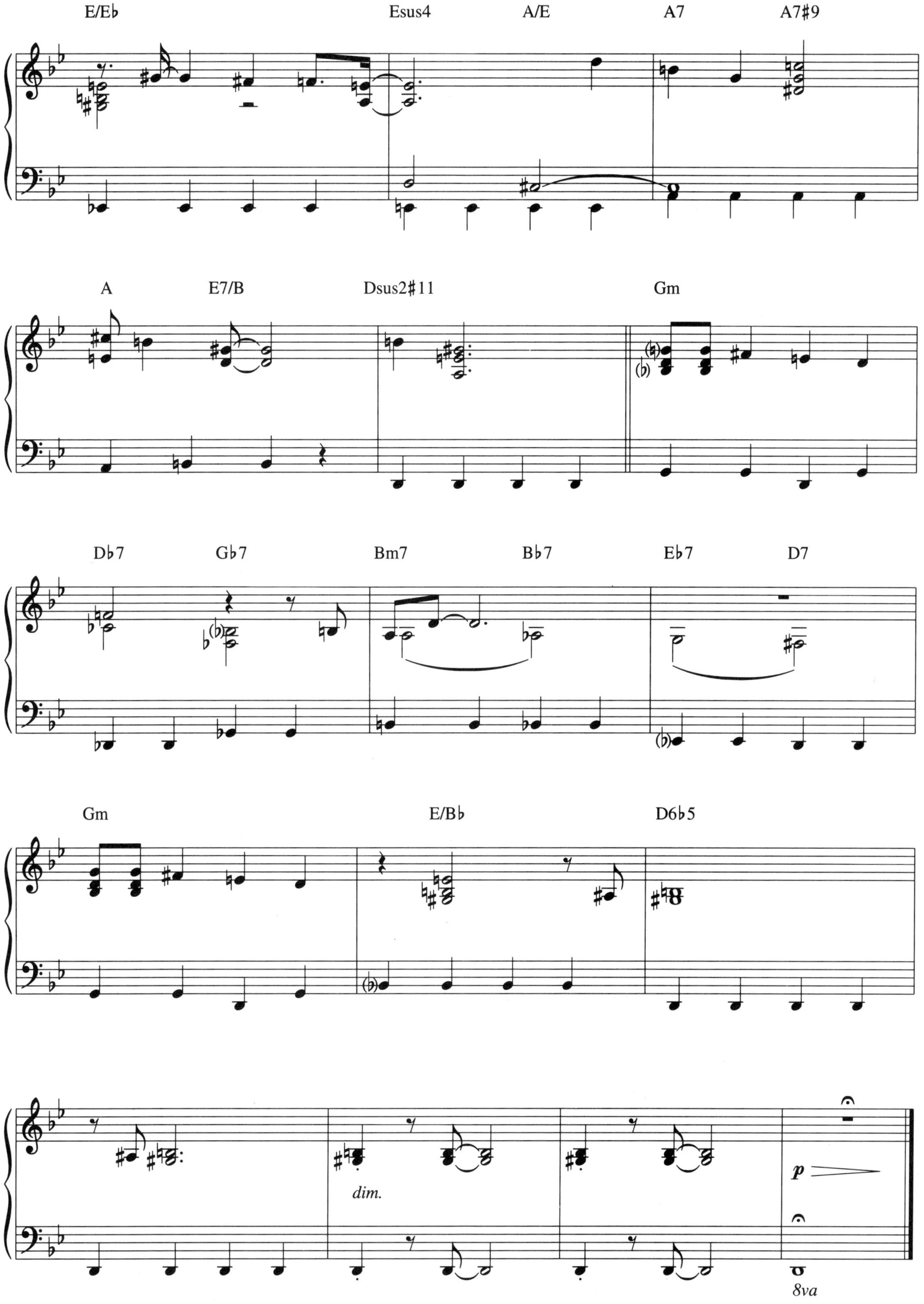
E/E♭
Esus4
A/E
A7
A7♯9
A
E7/B
Dsus2♯11
Gm
D♭7
G♭7
Bm7
B♭7
E♭7
D7
Gm
E/B♭
D6♭5
dim.
p
8va

Oop Bop Sh' Bam

by Dizzy Gillespie, Walter Fuller and Jay Roberts

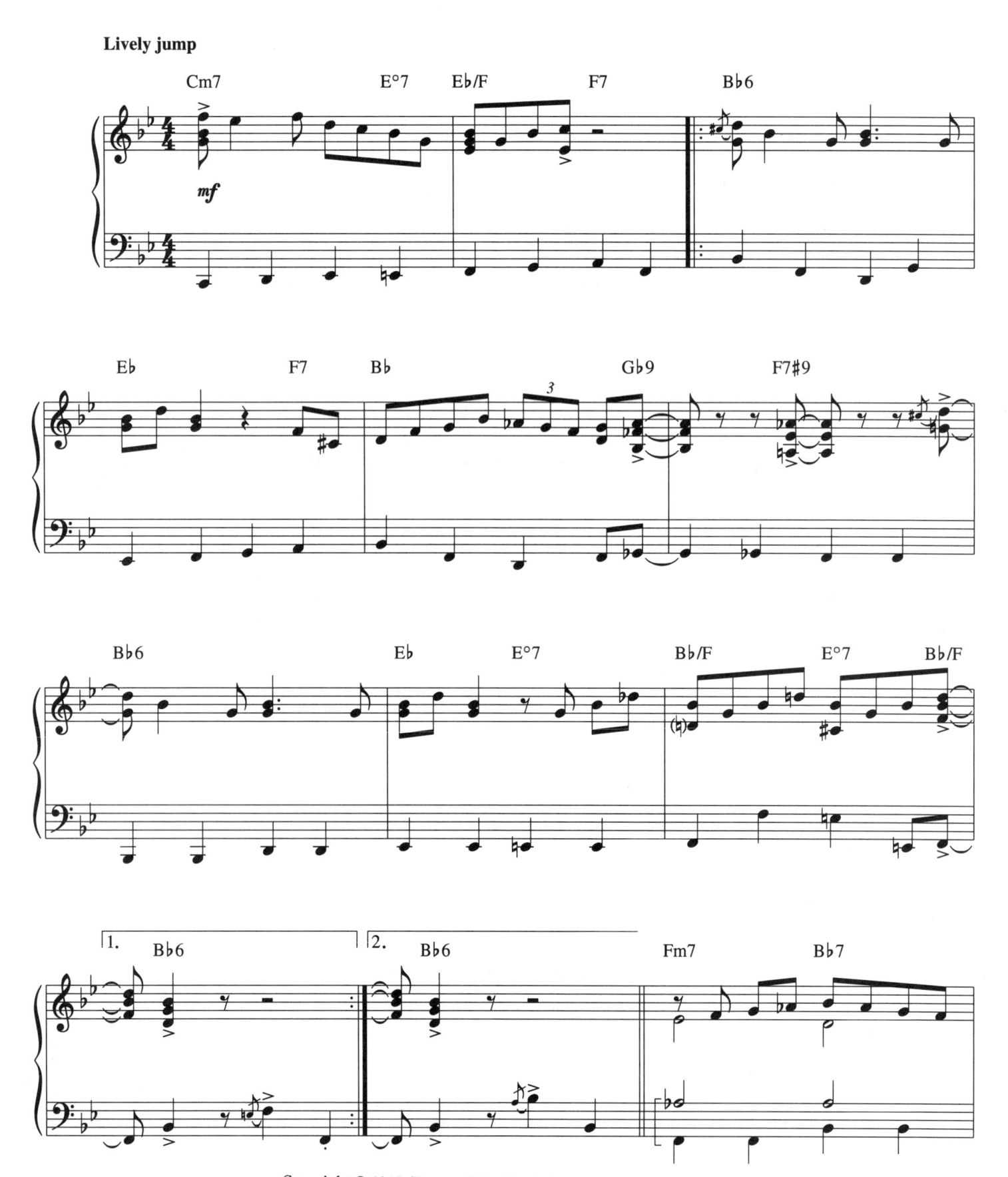

Lively jump

Copyright © 1946 (Renewed) by Music Sales Corporation (ASCAP)
International Copyright Secured. All Rights Reserved.

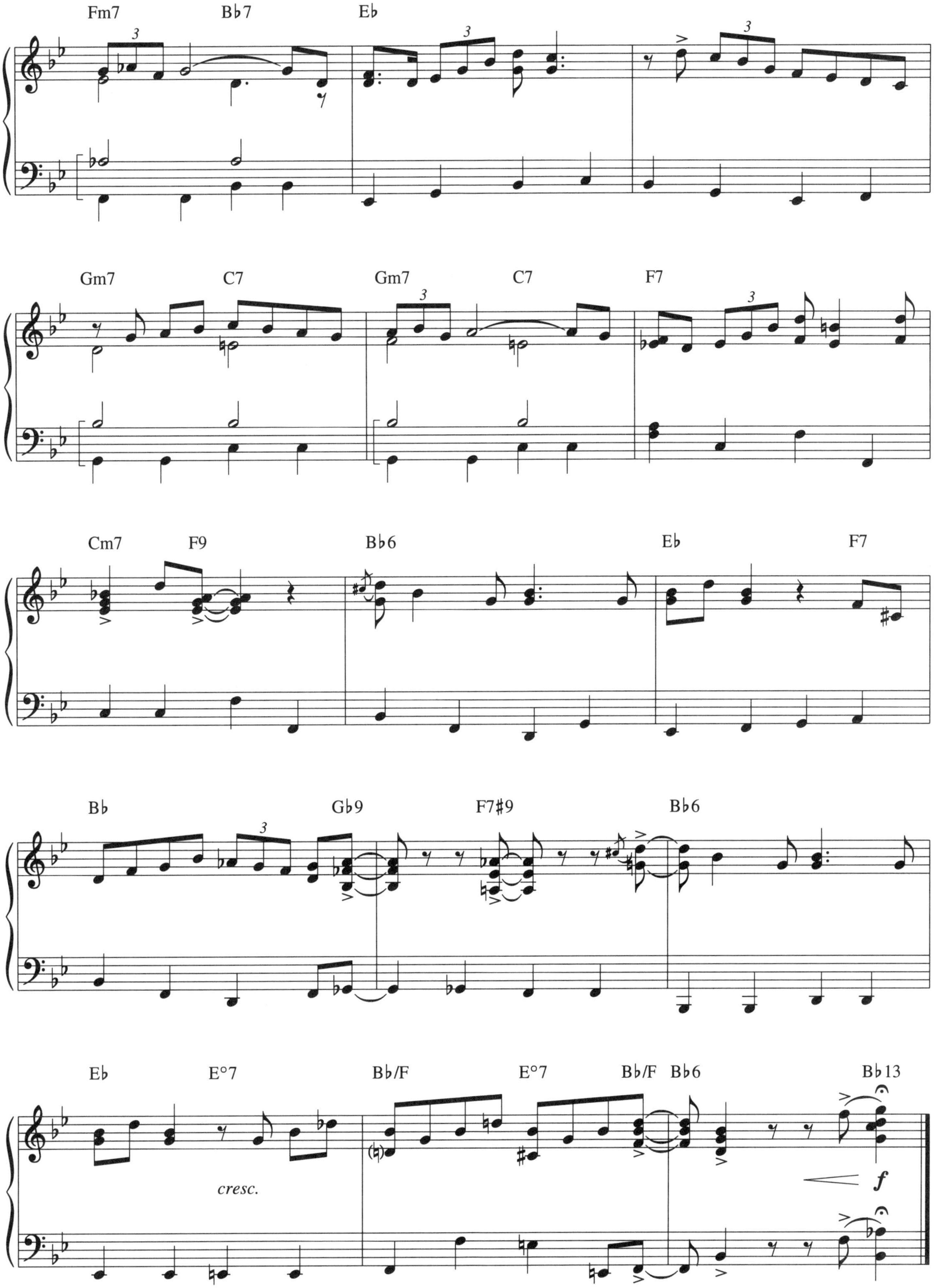
Fm7 Bb7 Eb
Gm7 C7 Gm7 C7 F7
Cm7 F9 Bb6 Eb F7
Bb Gb9 F7#9 Bb6
Eb E°7 Bb/F E°7 Bb/F Bb6 Bb13
cresc.
f

Lush Life

by Billy Strayhorn

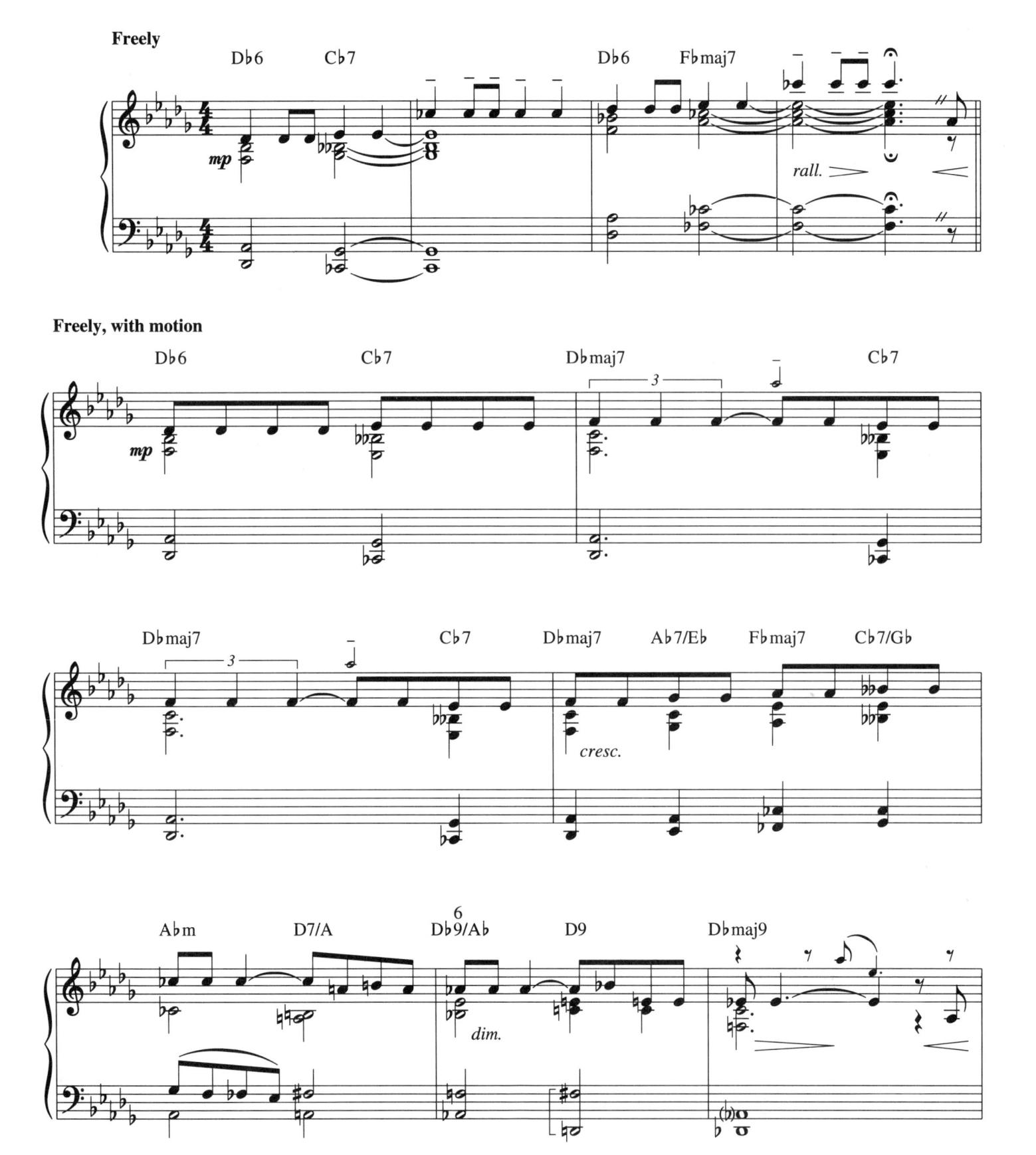

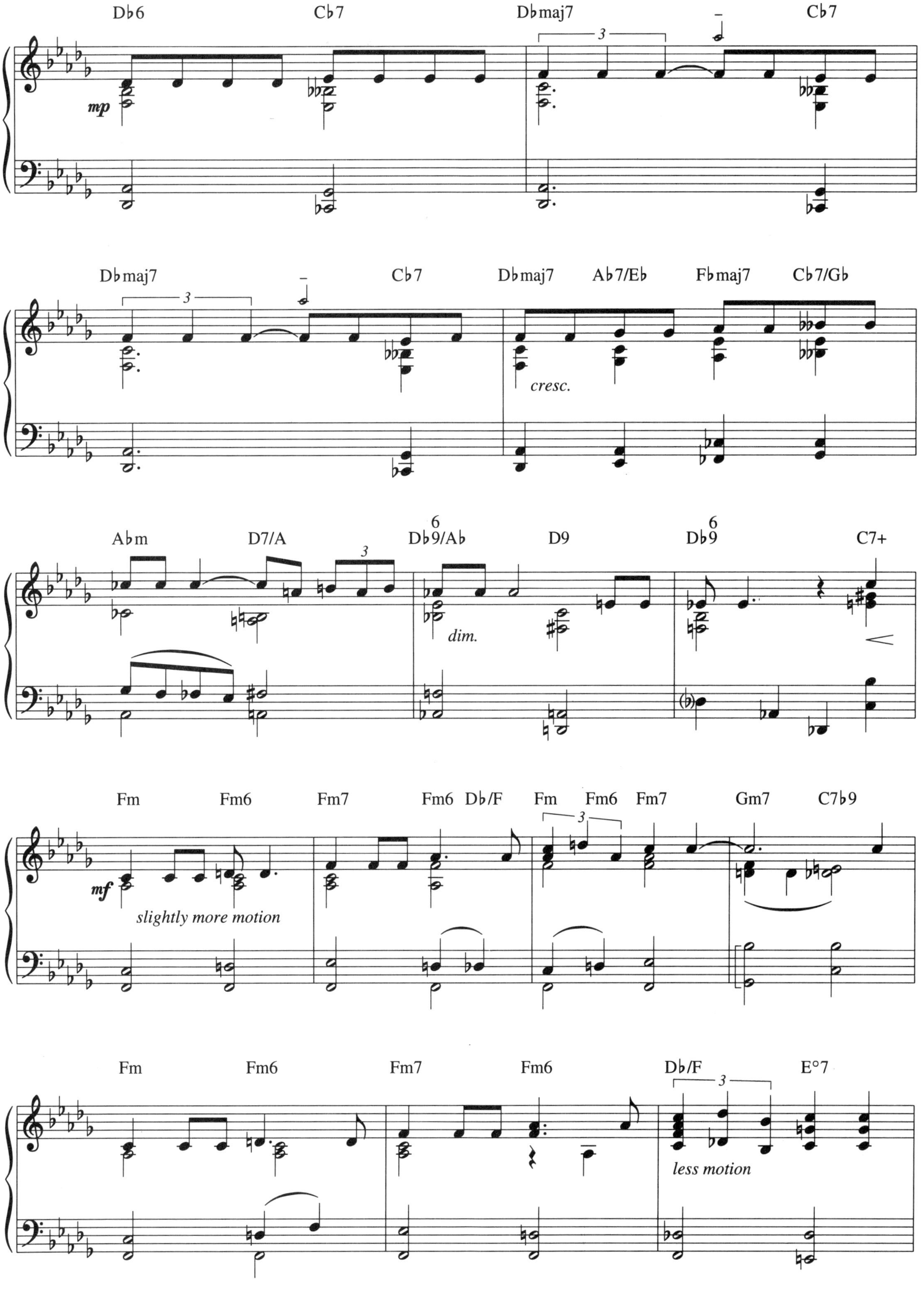
Db6 Cb7 Dbmaj7 Cb7
mp
Dbmaj7 Cb7 Dbmaj7 Ab7/Eb Fbmaj7 Cb7/Gb
cresc.
Abm D7/A Db9/Ab (6) D9 Db9 (6) C7+
dim.
Fm Fm6 Fm7 Fm6 Db/F Fm Fm6 Fm7 Gm7 C7b9
mf
slightly more motion
Fm Fm6 Fm7 Fm6 Db/F E°7
less motion

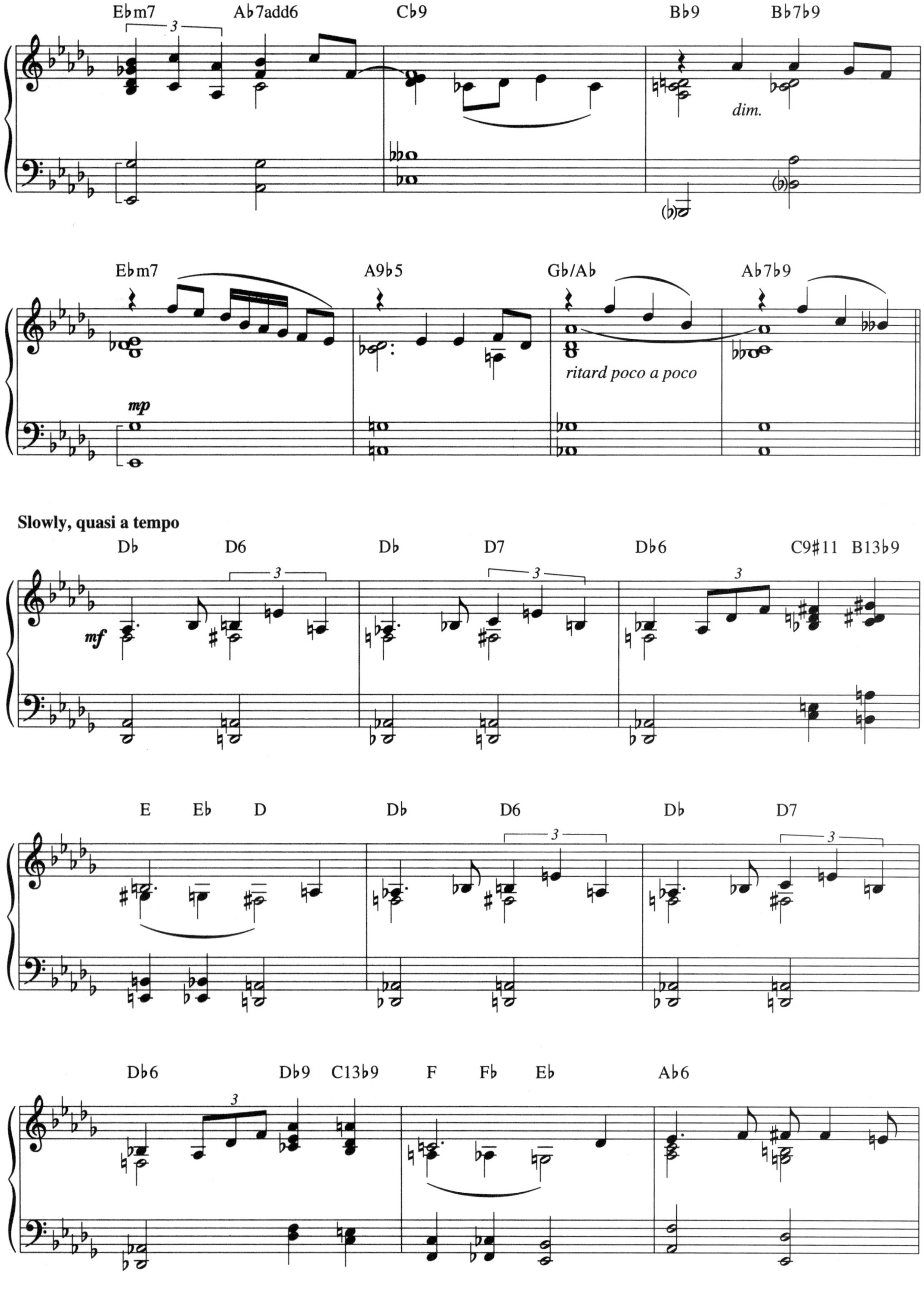
Ebm7 Ab7add6 Cb9 Bb9 Bb7b9
dim.
Ebm7 A9b5 Gb/Ab Ab7b9
mp
ritard poco a poco
Slowly, quasi a tempo
Db D6 Db D7 Db6 C9#11 B13b9
mf
E Eb D Db D6 Db D7
Db6 Db9 C13b9 F Fb Eb Ab6

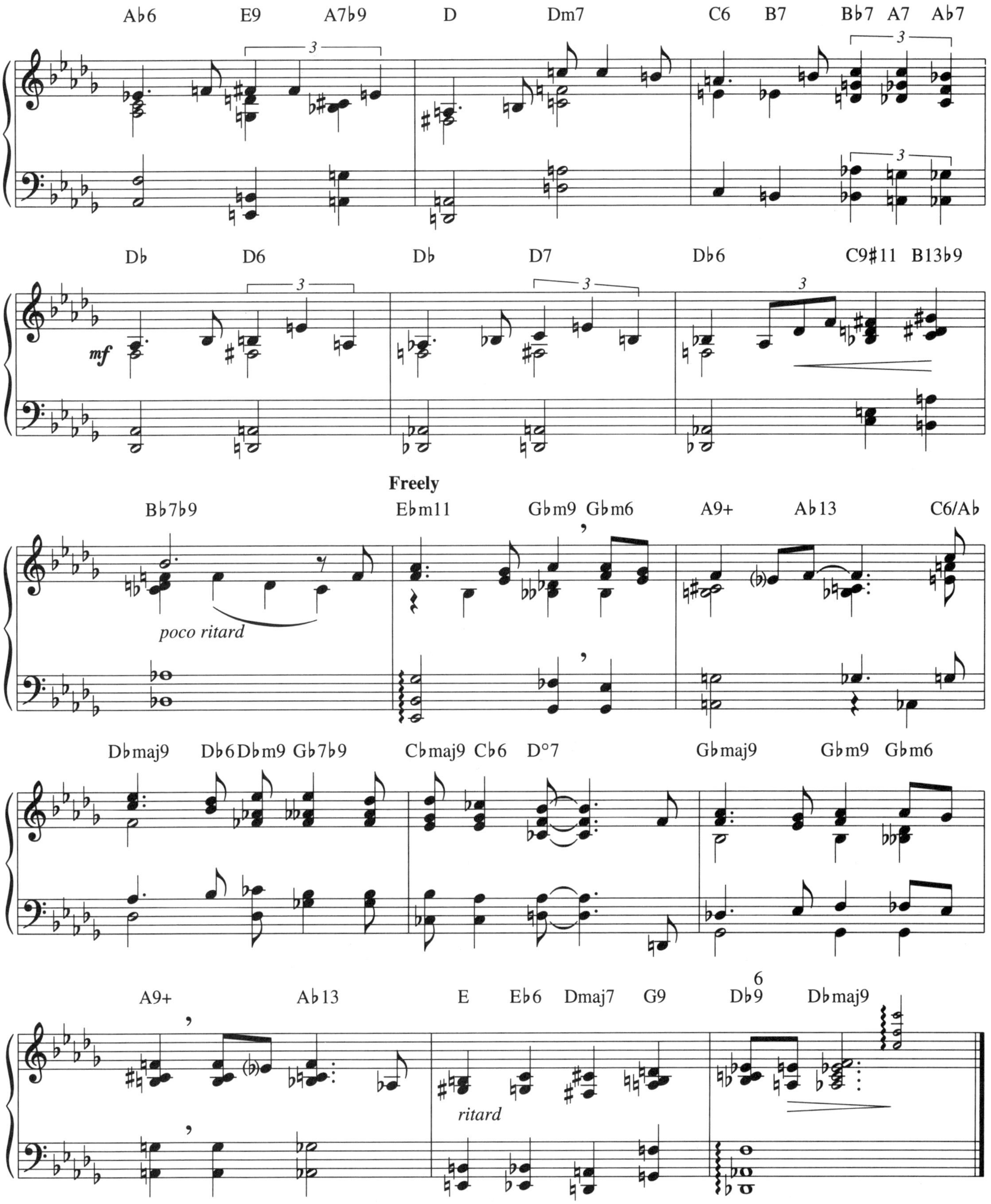
Ab6 E9 A7b9 D Dm7 C6 B7 Bb7 A7 Ab7
Db D6 Db D7 Db6 C9#11 B13b9
mf
Freely
Bb7b9 Ebm11 Gbm9 Gbm6 A9+ Ab13 C6/Ab
poco ritard
Dbmaj9 Db6 Dbm9 Gb7b9 Cbmaj9 Cb6 D°7 Gbmaj9 Gbm9 Gbm6
A9+ Ab13 E Eb6 Dmaj7 G9 Db9 6 Dbmaj9
ritard

Shaw Nuff

by Dizzy Gillespie and Charlie Parker

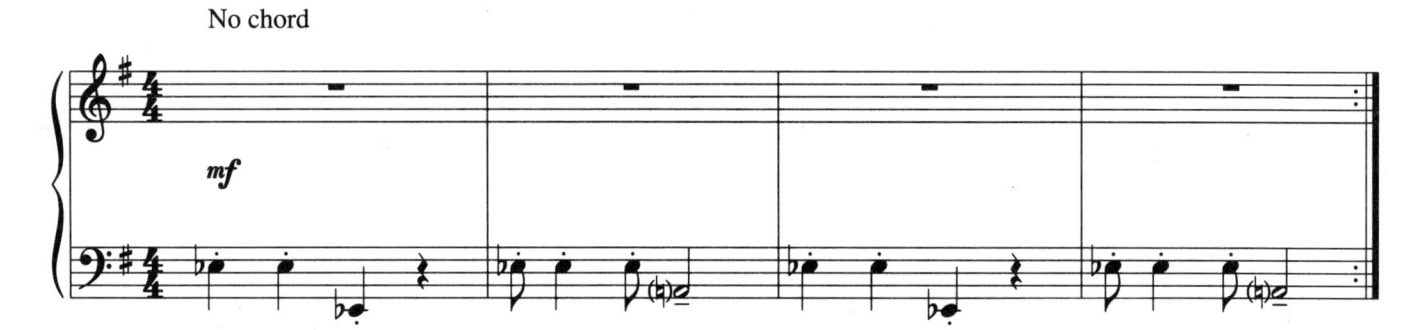

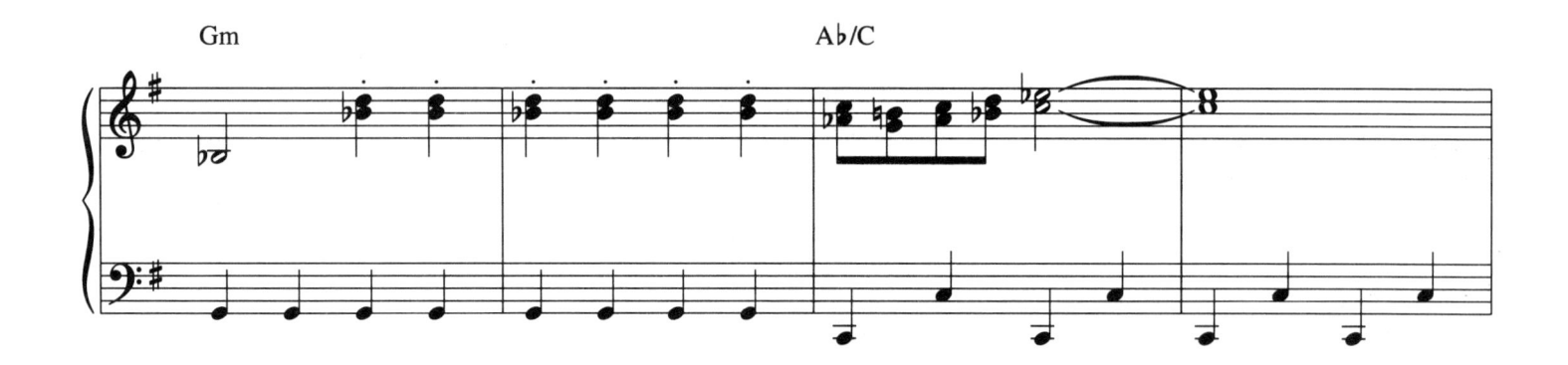

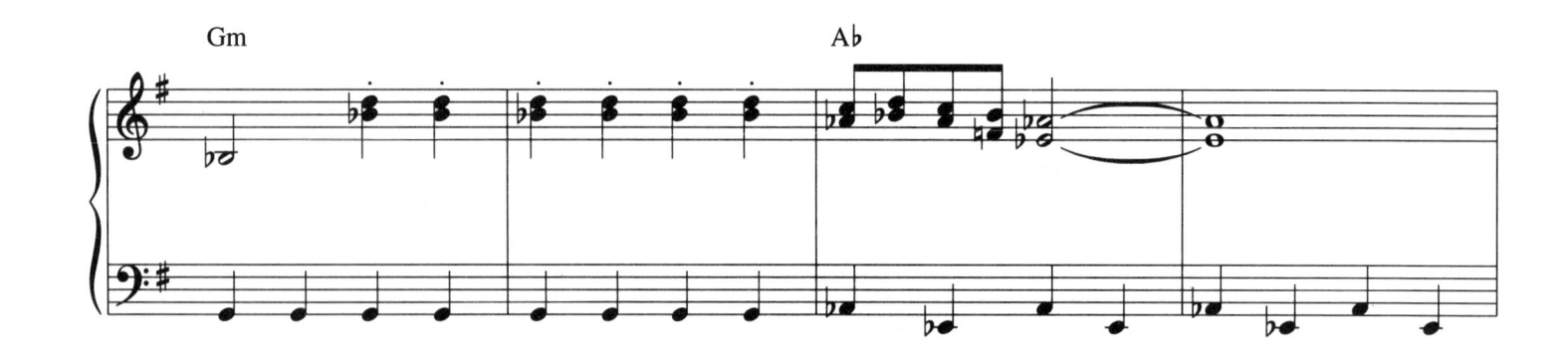

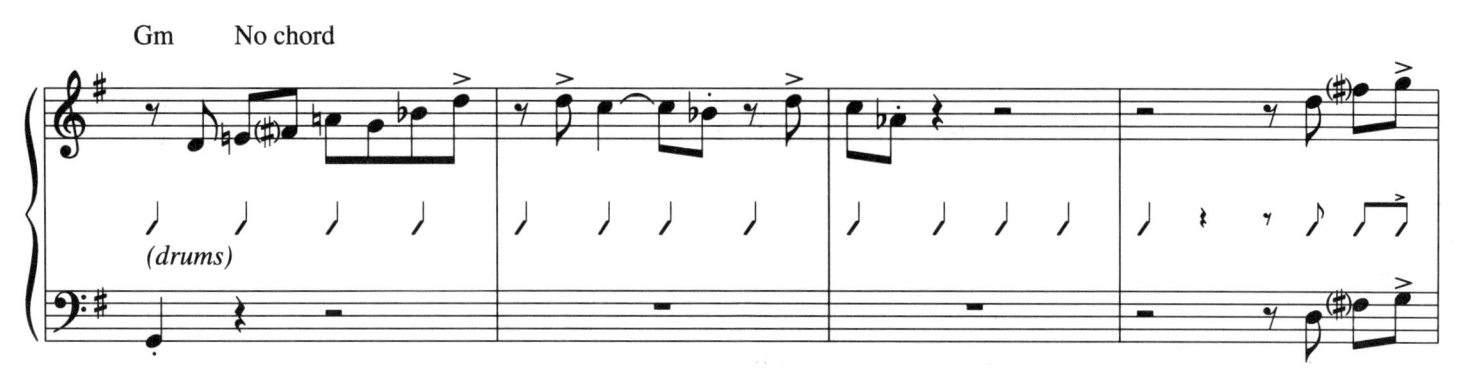

53

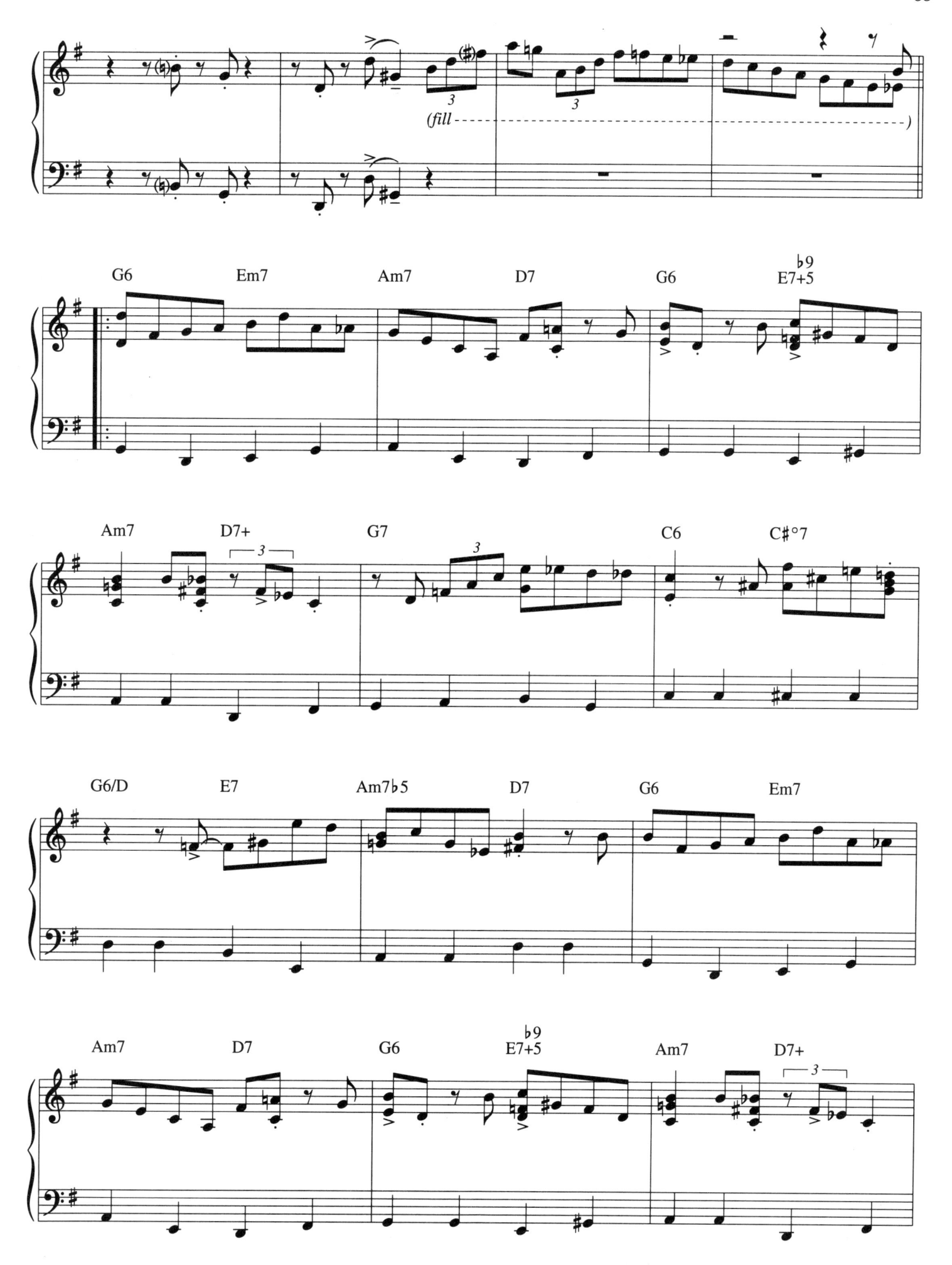

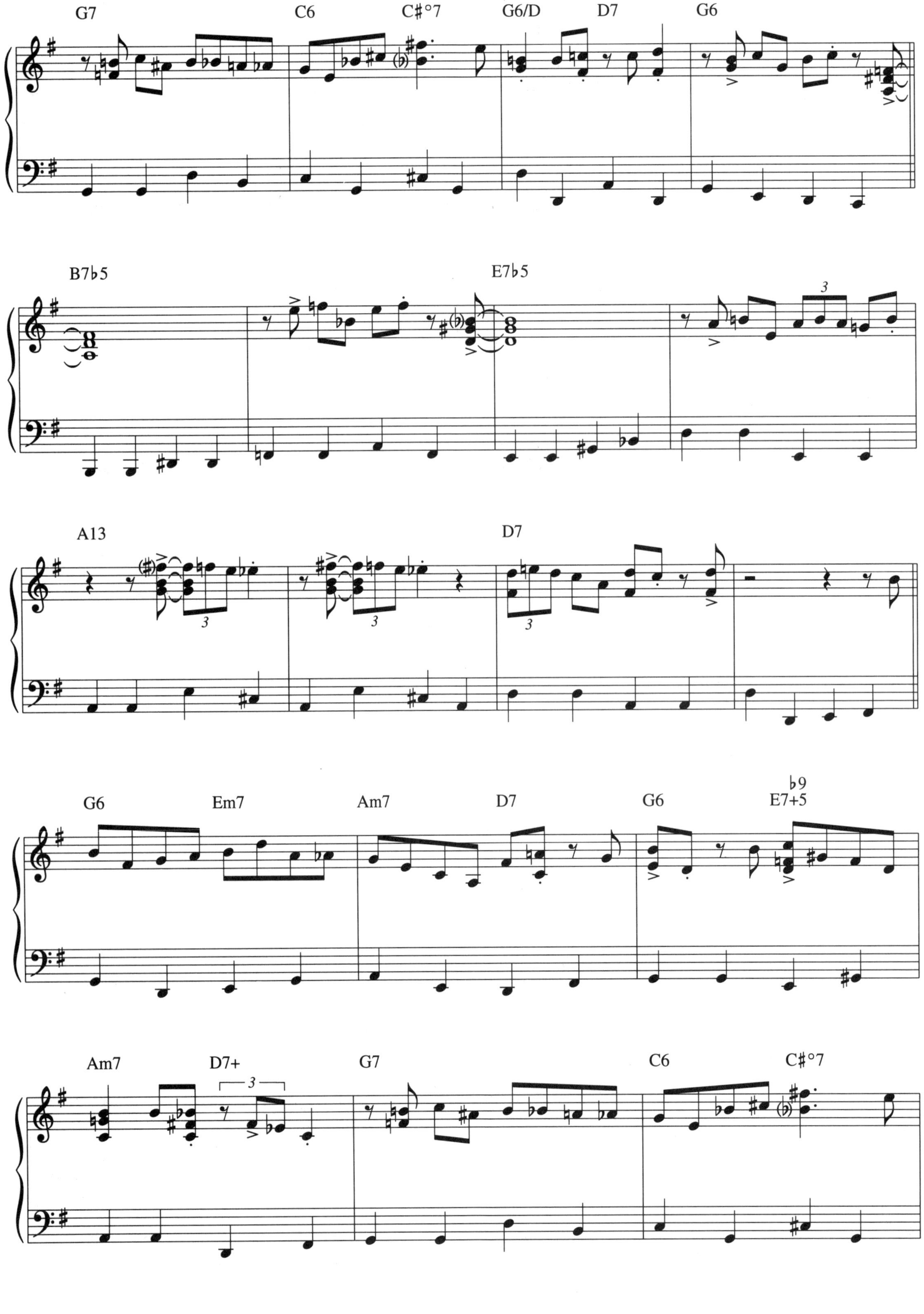
G7
C6
C♯°7
G6/D
D7
G6
B7♭5
E7♭5
A13
D7
G6
Em7
Am7
D7
G6
♭9
E7+5
Am7
D7+
G7
C6
C♯°7

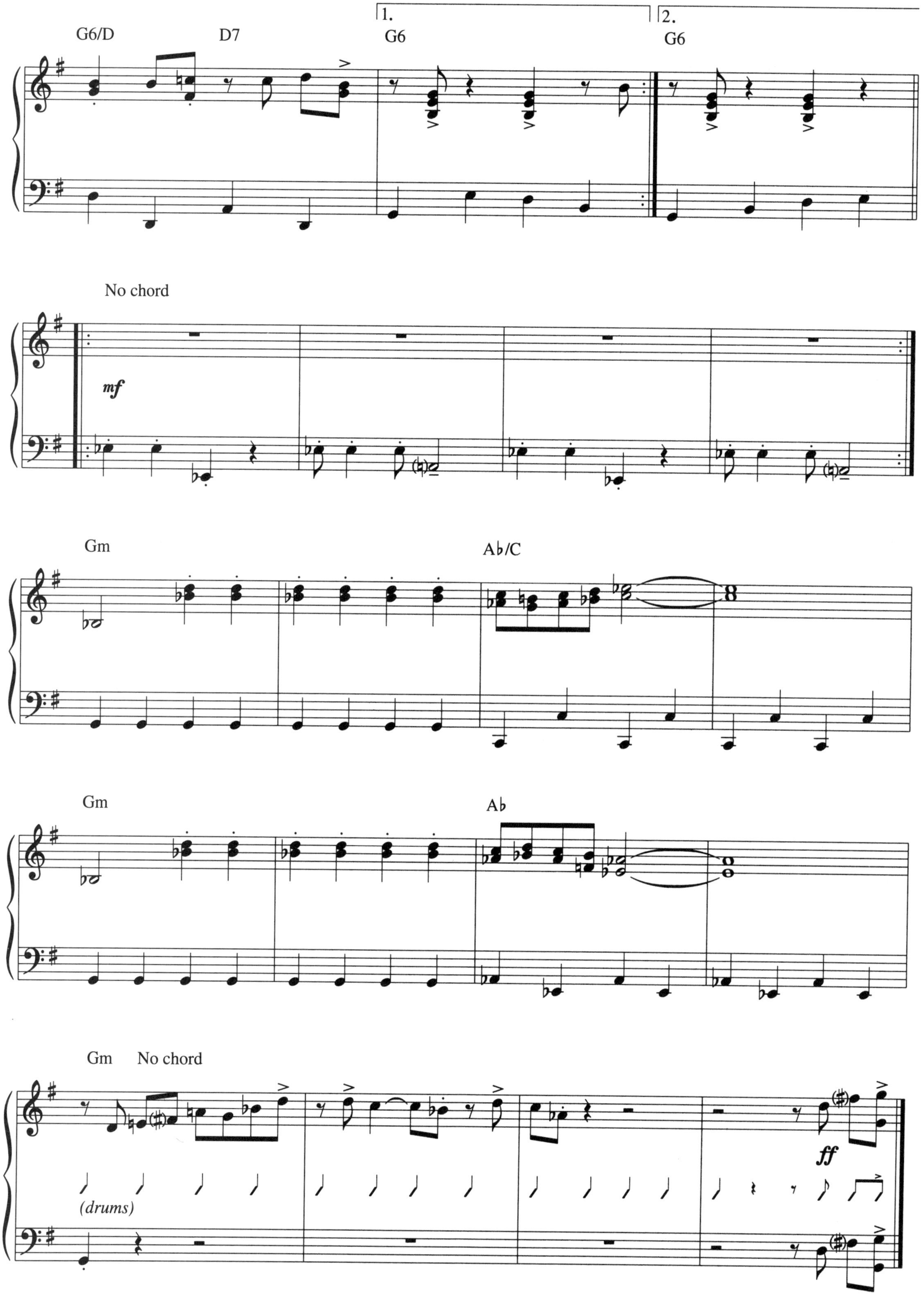

G6/D
D7
1.
G6
2.
G6
No chord
mf
Gm
A♭/C
Gm
A♭
Gm
No chord
(drums)
ff

Tempus Fugit

by Earl 'Bud' Powell

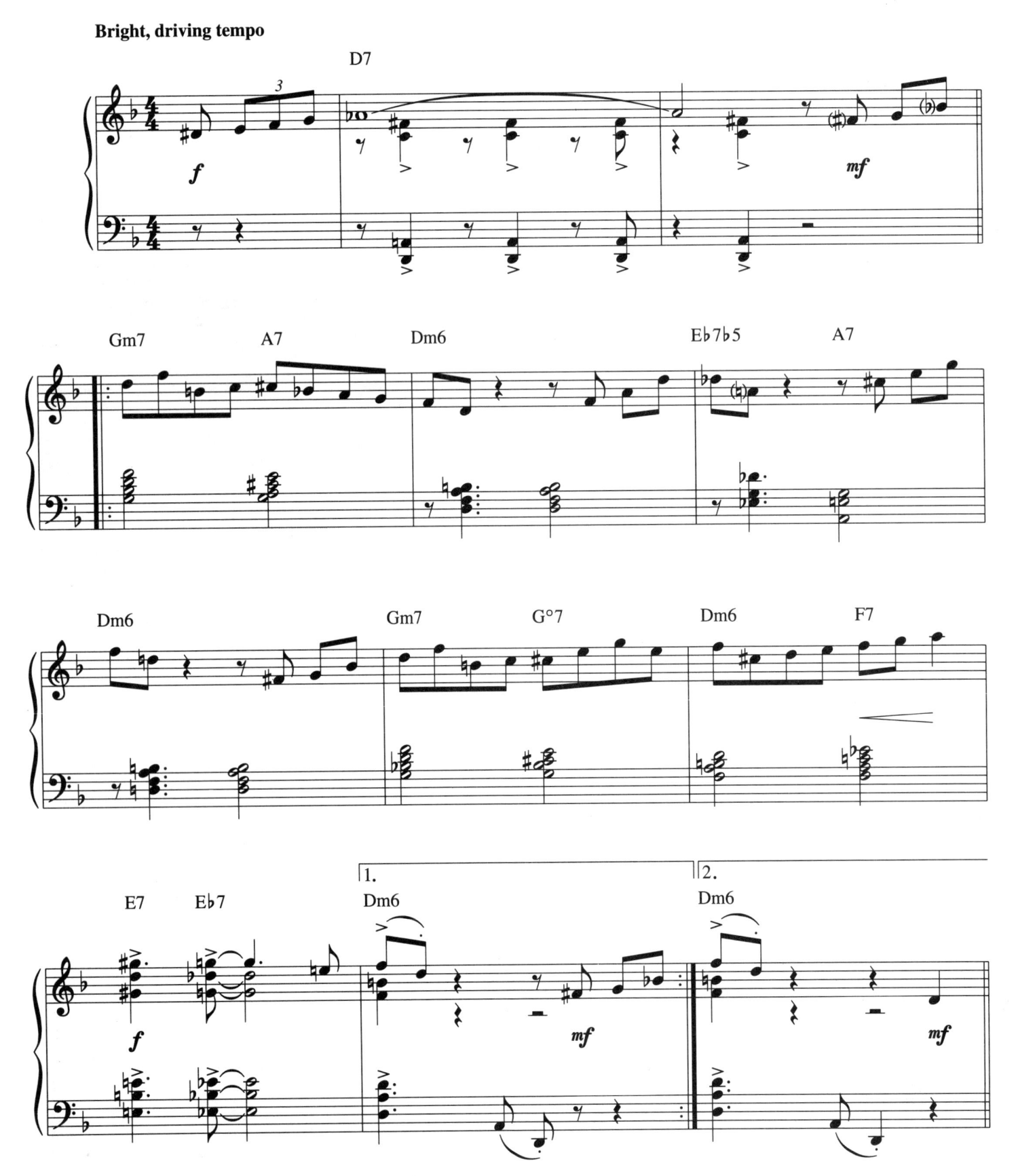

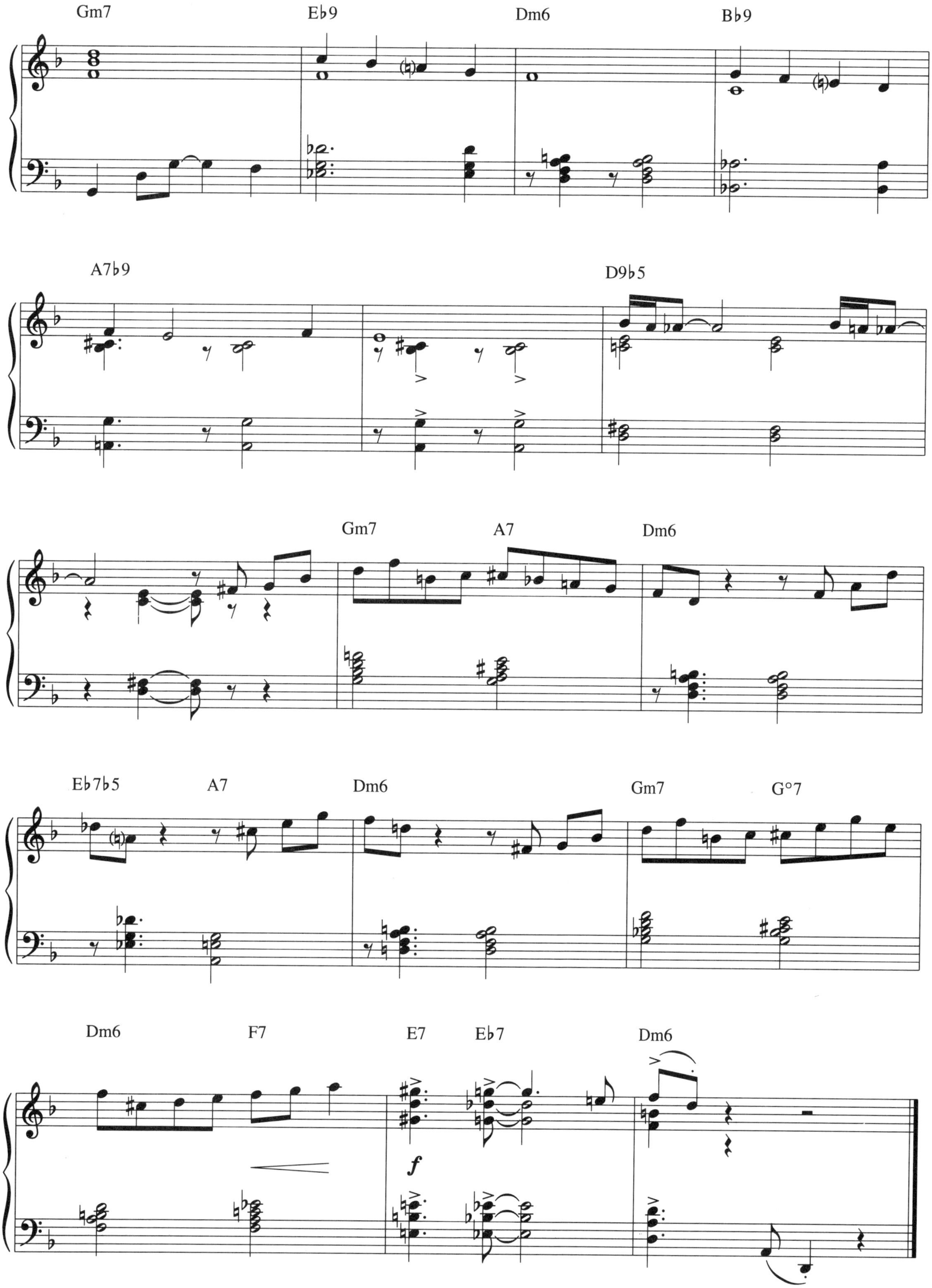
Gm7
E♭9
Dm6
B♭9
A7♭9
D9♭5
Gm7
A7
Dm6
E♭7♭5
A7
Dm6
Gm7
G°7
Dm6
F7
E7
E♭7
Dm6
f

Blood Count

by Billy Strayhorn

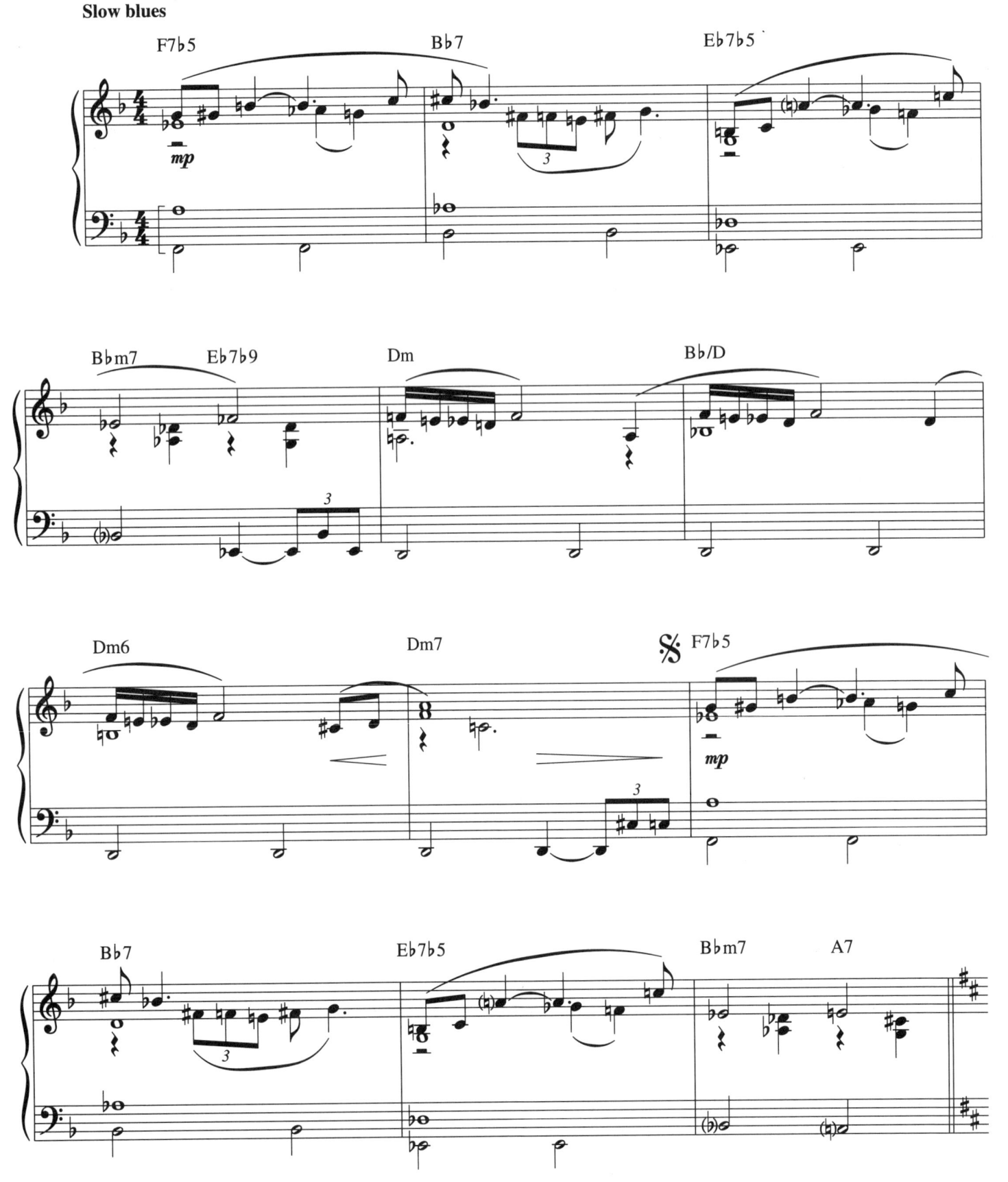

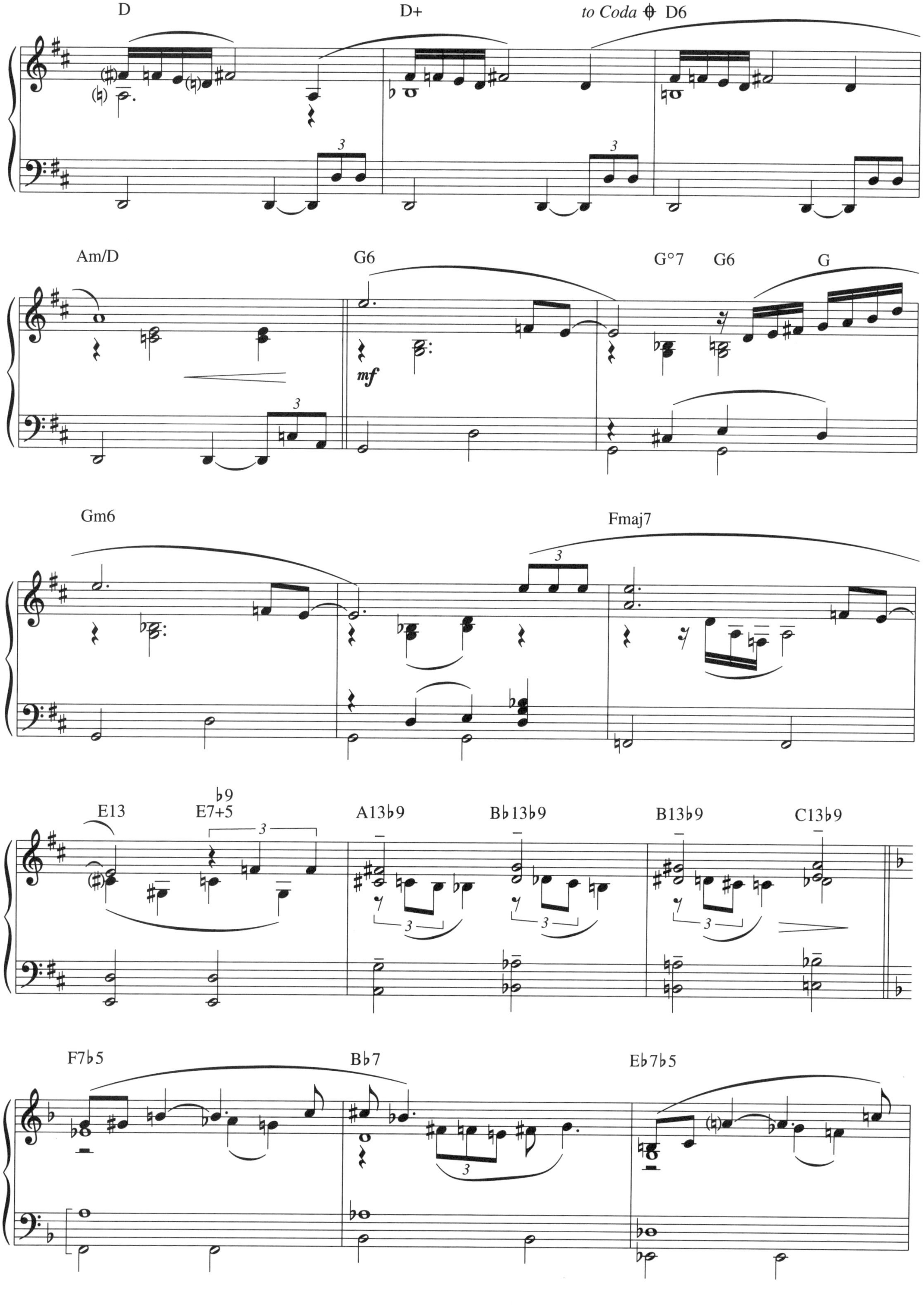
D
D+
to Coda
D6
Am/D
G6
G°7
G6
G
mf
Gm6
Fmaj7
E13
E7+5 ♭9
A13♭9
B♭13♭9
B13♭9
C13♭9
F7♭5
B♭7
E♭7♭5

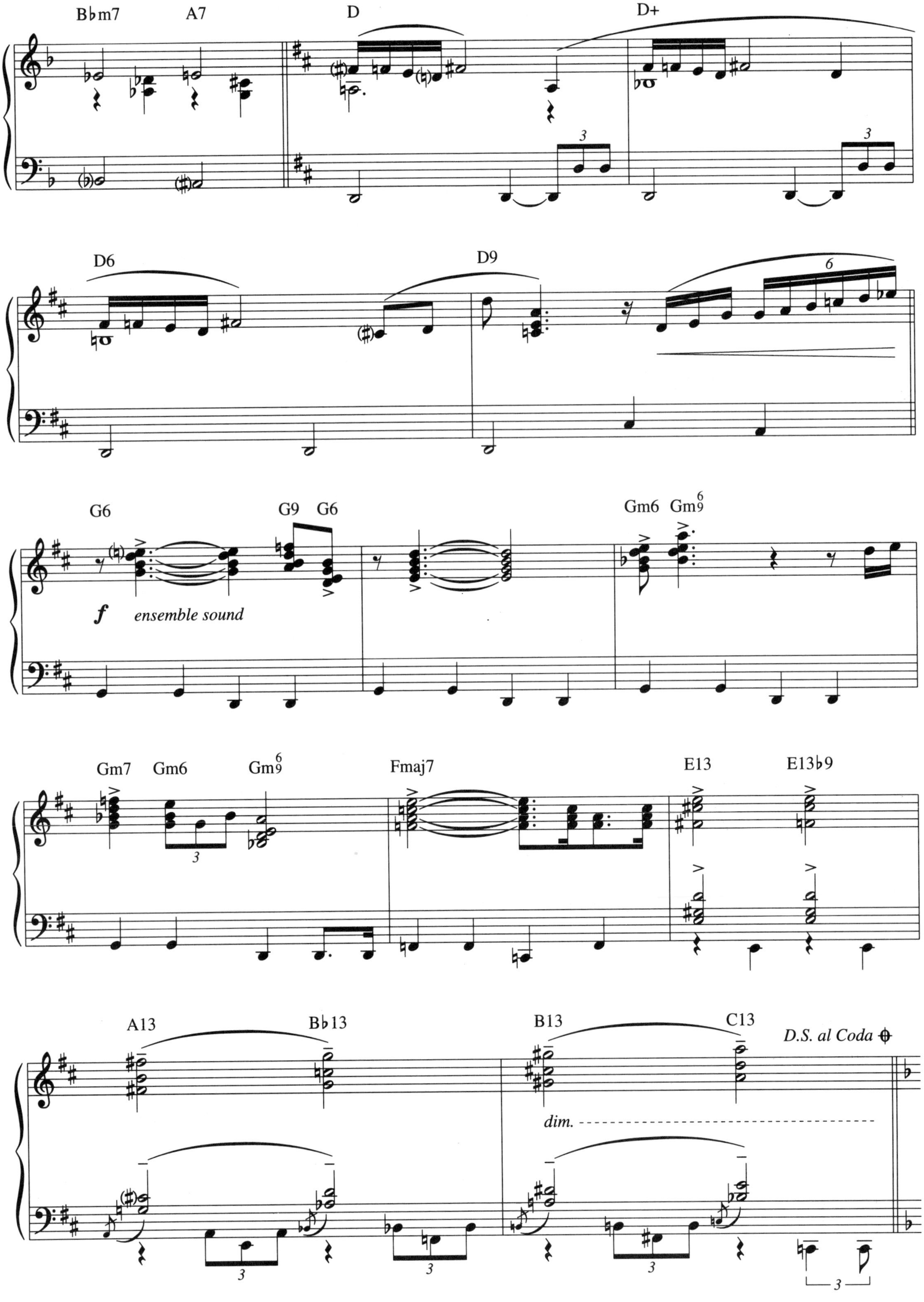
B♭m7
A7
D
D+
D6
D9
6
G6
G9
G6
f
ensemble sound
Gm6
Gm9 6
Gm7
Gm6
Gm9 6
Fmaj7
E13
E13♭9
A13
B♭13
B13
C13
D.S. al Coda
dim.
3

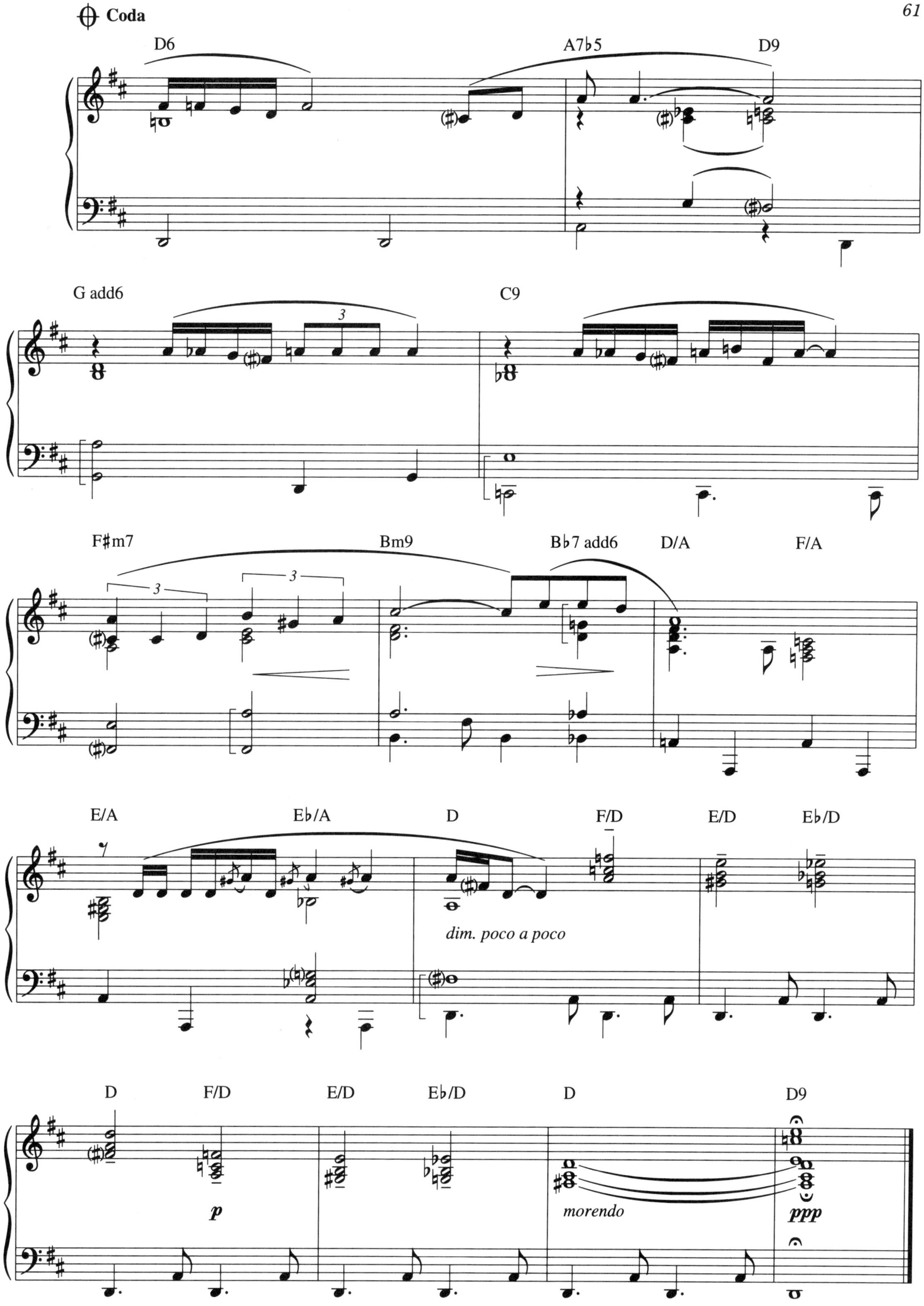
Coda
D6
A7♭5
D9
G add6
C9
F♯m7
Bm9
B♭7 add6
D/A
F/A
E/A
E♭/A
D
F/D
E/D
E♭/D
dim. poco a poco
D
F/D
E/D
E♭/D
D
D9
p
morendo
ppp

Jersey Bounce

by Robert Wright, Bobby Platter, Tiny Bradshaw and Ed Johnson

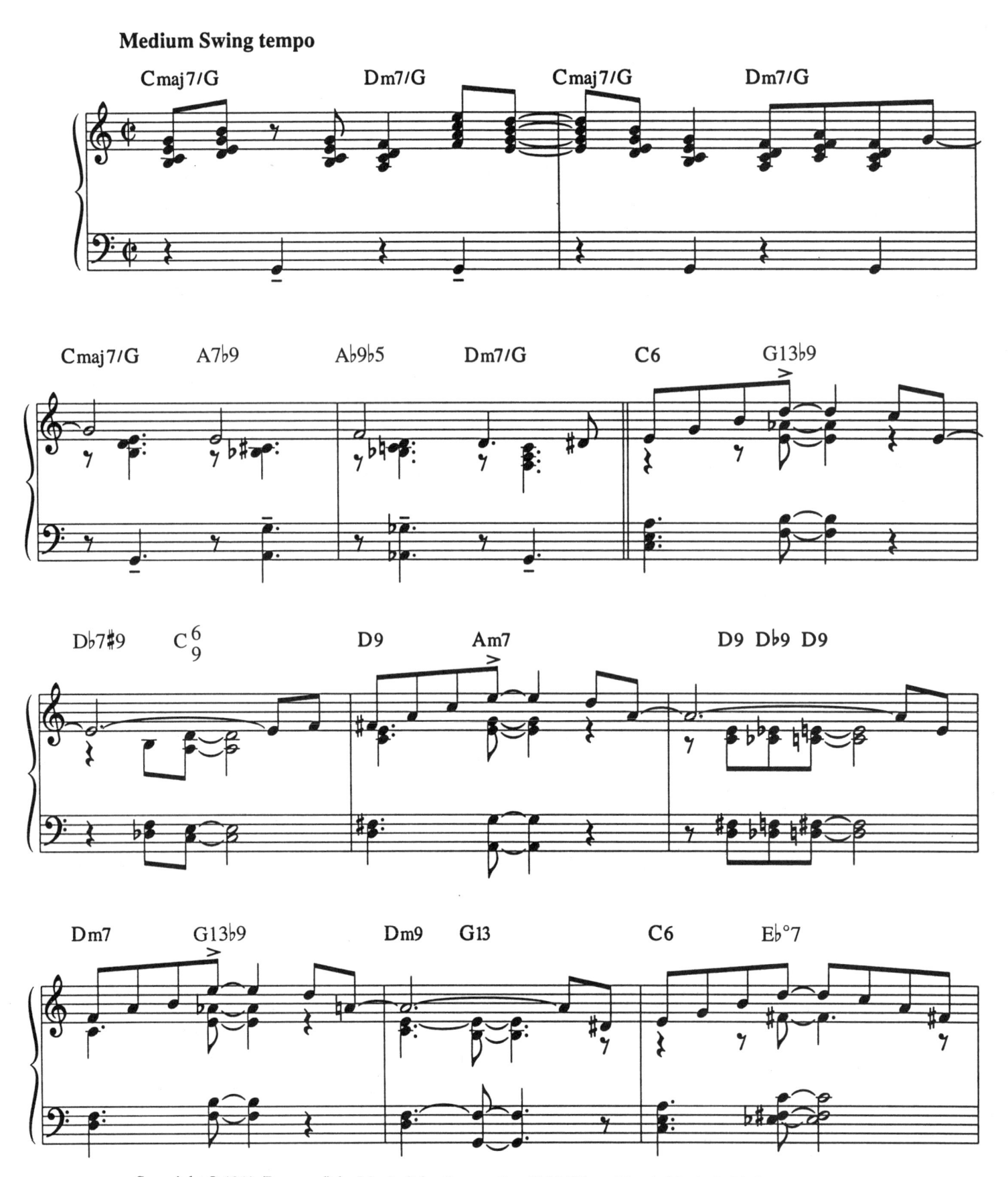

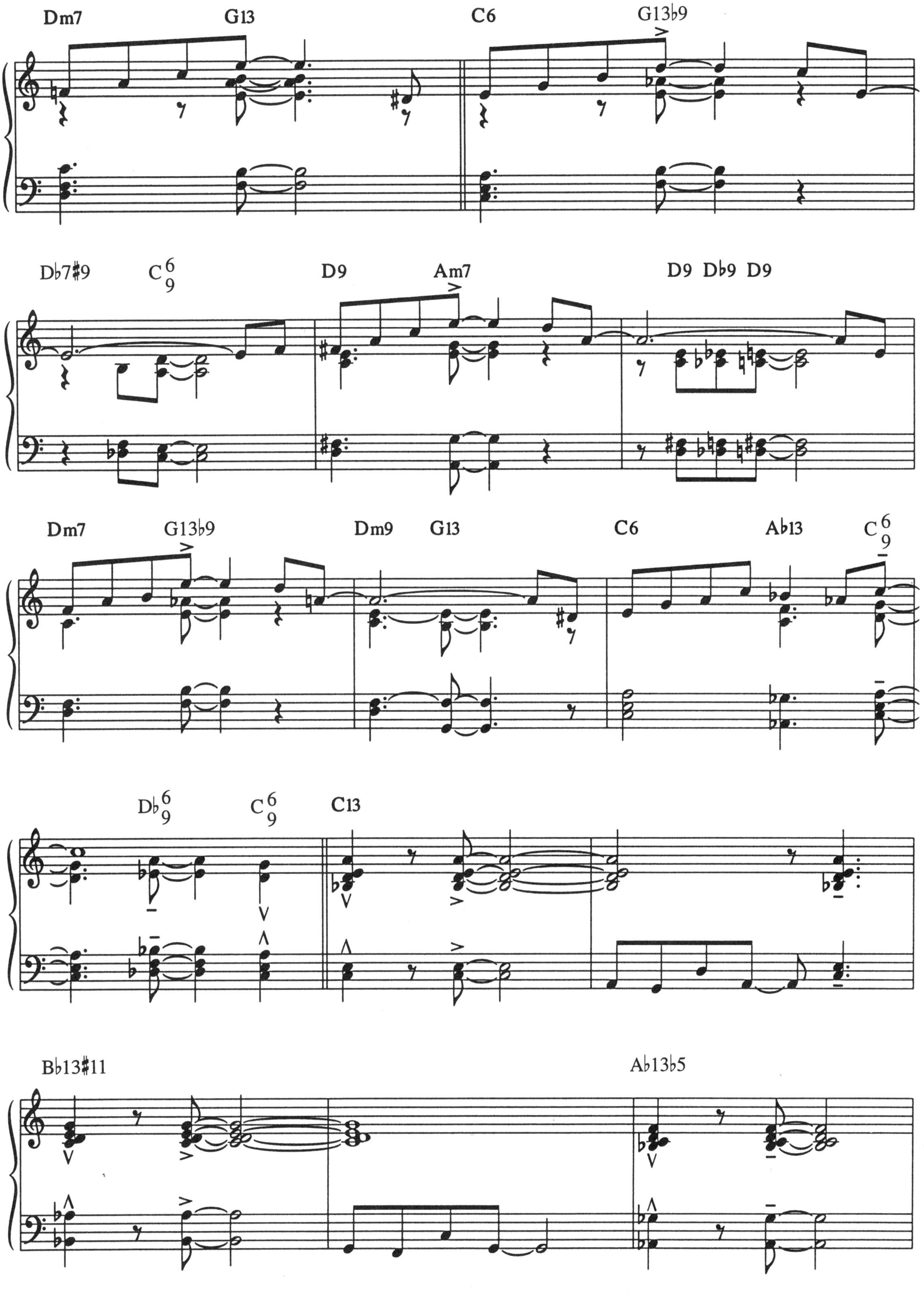
Dm7
G13
C6
G13♭9
D♭7♯9
C 6/9
D9
Am7
D9 D♭9 D9
Dm7
G13♭9
Dm9
G13
C6
A♭13
C 6/9
D♭ 6/9
C 6/9
C13
B♭13♯11
A♭13♭5

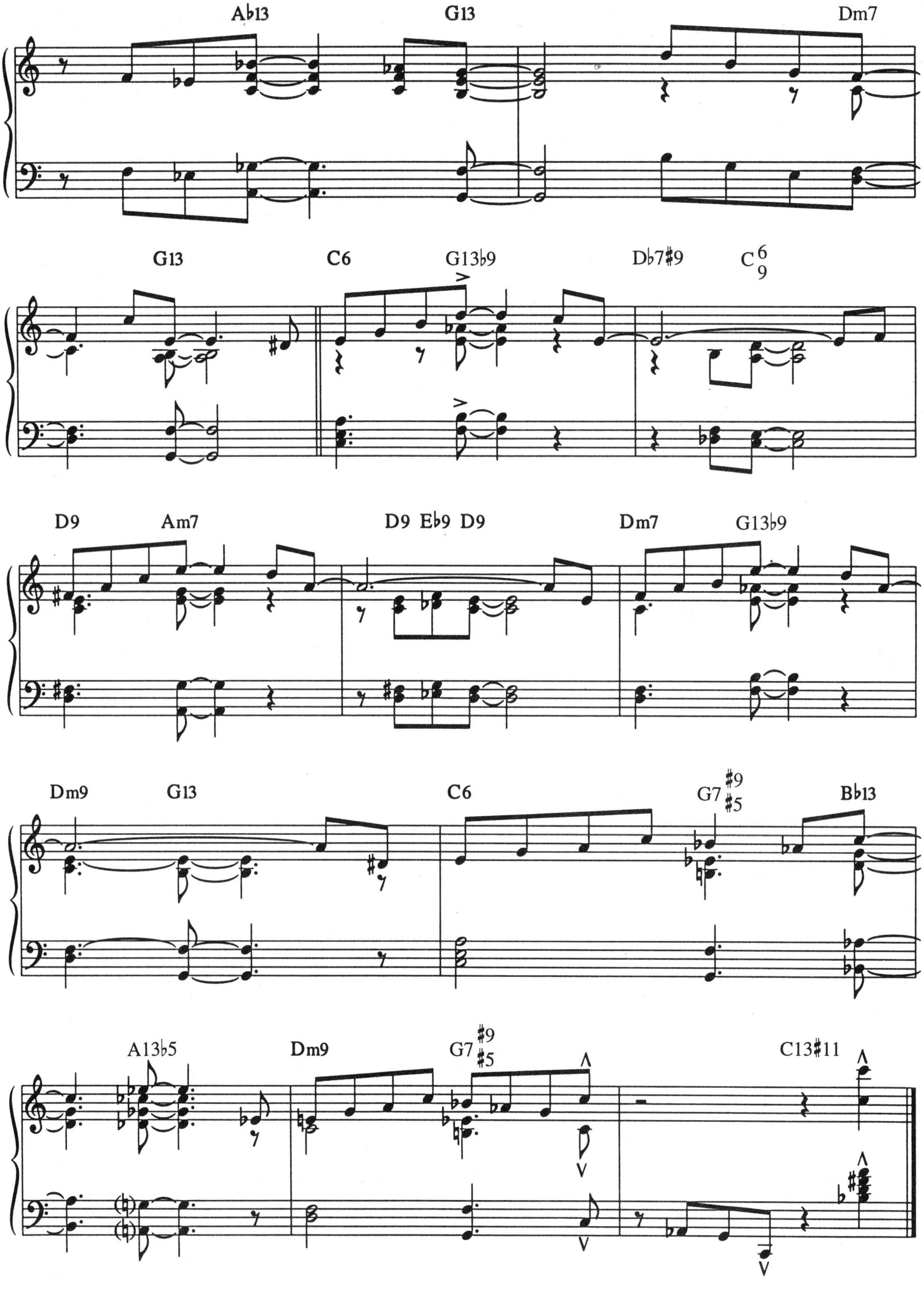
A♭13
G13
Dm7
G13
C6
G13♭9
D♭7♯9
C 6 9
D9
Am7
D9 E♭9 D9
Dm7
G13♭9
Dm9
G13
C6
G7 ♯9 ♯5
B♭13
A13♭5
Dm9
G7 ♯9 ♯5
C13♯11